Medical Intelligence Unit

Gene Therapy of Autoimmune Diseases

Gérald J. Prud'homme, M.D.
Department of Laboratory Medicine and Pathobiology
University of Toronto
St. Michael's Hospital
Toronto, Ontario, Canada

Landes Bioscience / Eurekah.com
Georgetown, Texas
U.S.A.

Kluwer Academic / Plenum Publishers
New York, New York
U.S.A.

Gene Therapy of Autoimmune Diseases

Medical Intelligence Unit

Landes Bioscience / Eurekah.com
Kluwer Academic / Plenum Publishers

Kluwer Academic / Plenum Publishers, 233 Spring Street, New York, New York, U.S.A. 10013
http://www.wkap.nl/

Please address all inquiries to the Publishers:
Landes Bioscience / Eurekah.com, 810 South Church Street
Georgetown, Texas, U.S.A. 78626
Phone: 512/ 863 7762; FAX: 512/ 863 0081
www.Eurekah.com
www.landesbioscience.com

Gene Therapy of Autoimmune Diseases, edited by Gérald J. Prud'homme, Landes / Kluwer dual imprint / Landes series: Medical Intelligence Unit

ISBN: 978-1-4419-3427-7 e-ISBN: 978-0-387-28670-9

Library of Congress Cataloging-in-Publication Data

Gene therapy of autoimmune diseases / [edited by] Gérald J. Prud'homme.
p. ; cm. -- (Medical intelligence unit)
Includes bibliographical references and index.

1. Autoimmune diseases--Gene therapy.
[DNLM: 1. Autoimmune Diseases--therapy. 2. Gene Therapy--methods. 3. Gene Targeting. 4. Gene Transfer Techniques. 5. Genetic Vectors. 6. Vaccines, DNA. WD 305 G329 2005] I. Prud'homme, Gérald J. II. Series: Medical intelligence unit (Unnumbered : 2003)
RC600.G45 2005
616.97'8042--dc22

2005005138

To my wife Danita, for providing essential inspiration
and support throughout my career.

CONTENTS

EDITOR

Gérald J. Prud'homme
Department of Laboratory Medicine and Pathobiology
University of Toronto
St. Michael's Hospital
Toronto, Ontario, Canada
Chapters 3, 7

CONTRIBUTORS

Natacha Bessis
UPRES EA-3408, Immunology
Université Paris 13
Bobigny, France
Chapter 5

Marie-Christophe Boissier
UPRES EA-3408
Université Paris 13
and
Service de Rhumatologie
Avicenne Hospital, AP-HP
Bobigny, France
Chapter 5

Erica Butti
Neuroimmunology Unit-DIBIT
Department of Neurology
and Neurophysiology
San Raffaele Scientific Institute
Milan, Italy
Chapter 1

Yigang Chang
Division of Immunogenetics
Children's Hospital of Pittsburgh
Pittsburgh University
Pittsburgh, Pennsylvania, U.S.A.
Chapter 7

Moustapha El-Amine
Iomai Corporation
Gaithersburg, Maryland, U.S.A.
Chapter 6

Roberto Furlan
Neuroimmunology Unit-DIBIT
Department of Neurology
and Neurophysiology
San Raffaele Scientific Institute
Milan, Italy
Chapter 1

Nick Giannoukakis
Department of Pathology
University of Pittsburgh School
of Medicine
Diabetes Institute
Rangos Research Center
Pittsburgh, Pennsylvania, U.S.A.
Chapter 2

Yelena Glinka
Department of Laboratory Medicine
and Pathobiology
St. Michael's Hospital
University of Toronto
Toronto, Ontario, Canada
Chapter 7

Justin M. Johnson
Department of Immunology
Lerner Research Institute
The Cleveland Clinic Foundation
Cleveland, Ohio, U.S.A.
Chapter 4

Xiaoying Li
Biomedical Research Center
University of British Columbia
Vancouver, British Columbia, Canada
Chapter 7

Mary Litzinger
Department of Immunology
Americcan Red Cross
Jerome Holland Laboratory
Rockville, Maryland
and
Department of Immunology
George Washington University
Medical Center
Washington, D.C., U.S.A.
Chapter 6

Gianvito Martino
Neuroimmunology Unit-DIBIT
Department of Neurology
and Neurophysiology
San Raffaele Scientific Institute
Milan, Italy
Chapter 1

Marco E.F. Melo
Department of Immunology
Americcan Red Cross
Jerome Holland Laboratory
Rockville, Maryland
and
Department of Immunology
George Washington University
Medical Center
Washington, D.C., U.S.A.
Chapter 6

Ciriaco A. Piccirillo
Department of Microbiology
and Immunology
McGill University
Montreal, Quebec, Canada
Chapter 3

Jon D. Piganelli
Department of Pediatrics
Diabetes Institute
University of Pittsburgh School
of Medicine
Pittsburgh, Pennsylvania, U.S.A.
Chapter 2

Stefano Pluchino
Neuroimmunology Unit-DIBIT
Department of Neurology
and Neurophysiology
San Raffaele Scientific Institute
Milan, Italy
Chapter 1

David W. Scott
Department of Immunology
Americcan Red Cross
Jerome Holland Laboratory
Rockville, Maryland
and
Department of Immunology
George Washington University
Medical Center
Washington, D.C., U.S.A.
Chapter 6

Argyrios N. Theofilopoulos
Department of Immunology
The Scripps Research Institute
La Jolla, California, U.S.A.
Chapter 3

Massimo Trucco
Department of Pediatrics
Diabetes Institute, Division
of Immunogenetics
University of Pittsburgh School
of Medicine
Pittsburgh, Pennsylvania, U.S.A.
Chapter 2

Vincent K. Tuohy
Department of Immunology
Lerner Research Institute
The Cleveland Clinic Foundation
Cleveland, Ohio, U.S.A.
Chapter 4

PREFACE

Autoimmune diseases such as type 1 diabetes (T1D), multiple sclerosis (MS), autoimmune thyroiditis, rheumatoid arthritis (RA) and systemic lupus erythematosus (SLE), to name a few, are common as a group and cause considerable morbidity in the population. In addition, there are numerous inflammatory disorders of unclear etiology, including various forms of arthritis, vasculitis, glomerulonephritis, pneumonitis, carditis, dermatitis and inflammatory bowel disease. Autoimmune/inflammatory diseases are hard to treat and can lead to premature death because current therapies are generally neither completely effective nor curative. Therapy has been slow to evolve, despite phenomenal advances in our understanding of immune mechanisms. Nevertheless, preclinical and clinical studies show that cytokine inhibitors (e.g., antibodies or soluble receptors) can be applied to the therapy of RA and other disorders. Unfortunately, it is difficult to apply these therapies clinically because large amounts of highly purified proteins are required and must be delivered repeatedly by parenteral routes. As therapeutic agents, most cytokines have pleiotropic activities, many unwanted, and tend to have serious toxic effects, while anticytokine agents can lead to depressed immunity and infection. There is also a rapidly growing literature documenting the protective effects of regulatory T cells and the regulatory cytokines that some subsets produce. However, cell-based therapies are even more demanding and expensive and must be individualized. In view of this, investigators have been looking for new approaches to immunotherapy, and gene therapy provides several interesting advantages.

Gene therapy can be applied in a systemic or tissue-localized fashion. It obviates the need for the frequent administration of protein drugs and allows relatively constant delivery of these proteins over long periods of time. Gene therapy can be accomplished with a wide variety of vectors, either viral or nonviral, although each method has its advantages and disadvantages. For instance, constant delivery of a cytokine at a low level can be effective and minimizes toxicity. Moreover, the therapeutic gene can be injected directly into the target tissue or, alternatively, carried by cells which have been transfected or transduced ex vivo. Thus, antigen-reactive T-cell lines or clones can carry an immunoregulatory gene to a specific target tissue such as the pancreas or central nervous system. Similarly, synovial cells can be altered by gene transfer ex vivo and returned to inflamed joints. Gene therapy also allows the delivery of a very wide variety of immune mediators, or inhibitors, which have well known biological properties. The development of conventional drugs duplicating these properties is difficult, extremely expensive and not always feasible.

An additional remarkable feature of immunogene therapy, as outlined in some chapters, is the ability to induce long-term tolerance. This can be accomplished by gene-based modification of antigen-presenting cells (notably B lymphocytes) or T cells, as well as the delivery of some immunoinhibitory molecules. Notably, DNA vaccination provides a new route for tolerogenic antigen therapy. These approaches are versatile and applicable to many autoimmune disorders.

Despite its promise, gene therapy of immunological diseases has not found its way into the clinic to any extent. To achieve this goal there are significant questions to resolve involving safety, as well as the persistence and regulation of gene expression. For instance, insulin gene therapy of T1D poses a formidable challenge because production of this hormone must be tightly regulated on a continuous basis. In this case, and other diseases where irreversible cell loss has occurred, gene therapy might be combined with transplantation (e.g., of islets of Langerhans) or stem cell therapy. Similarly, in vivo or ex vivo gene transfer might be applied to stimulate tissue regeneration. The chronic nature of many autoimmune diseases represents a serious impediment since we must design therapies that are effective over very long periods of time. Obviously, immunity against the vector, and any vector-related pathology, are not desirable.

The authors of this book have pioneered the application of gene therapy for autoimmune diseases, and they review many successful approaches. They describe how autoaggressive immune responses can be prevented, diminished or blocked, and outline the best avenues for the future. The relevance of the recently revived regulatory (suppressor) T cells is addressed, and some new (exciting) agents such as siRNA are introduced. Each author approaches the topic from a different perspective, although there is inevitable overlap, and it is hoped that this will give the reader a comprehensive view of the evolution and potential of this field.

Gérald J. Prud'homme, MD
November 29, 2004
Toronto, Canada

Chapter 1

Gene Therapy Approaches for Autoimmune Diseases of the Central Nervous System and Other Tissues

Roberto Furlan,* Erica Butti, Stefano Pluchino and Gianvito Martino

Introduction

Autoimmune disorders are the result of an aberrant immune reaction against self-components of the organism. Genetic traits, conferring predisposition to break immunological tolerance to self-antigens, are thought to concur, together with environmental factors, in the aetiology of this large, growing family of diseases. The different nosological entities classified within the autoimmune family share some clinical and immunological features: (i) females are more affected than males, with the notable exception of type I diabetes (IDDM) that, however, becomes clinically evident before completion of the sexual development; (ii) disease course is usually unpredictable—from benign cases to malignant overaggressive situations—making prognostic evaluation, at an individual level, very difficult; and, (iii) an immunological mechanism sustained by Th1-polarized $CD4^+$ cells is thought to be responsible for the auto-aggressive reaction.

Etiological treatments for diseases affecting millions of patients worldwide–such as multiple sclerosis (MS), rheumatoid arthritis (RA), IDDM, Hashimoto thyroiditis—are still lacking and current available therapies do not control satisfactorily the disease evolution. Current therapeutic strategies for all autoimmune diseases rely on immunosuppressive and/or symptomatic therapies that preserve only partially the patients' quality of life. Thus, new technological approaches to these disorders should be developed.

Gene Therapy of Autoimmune Disorders

General Principles

Gene therapy has been so far widely applied only to experimental models of autoimmune disorders. To our knowledge, only one human phase I trial for RA has been already completed.[1]

*Roberto Furlan—Department of Neurology and Neurophysiology, Neuroimmunology Unit-DIBIT, San Raffaele Scientific Instituite, Via Olgettina 58, 20132 Milan, Italy. Email: furlan.roberto@hsr.it

Gene Therapy of Autoimmune Disease, edited by Gérald J. Prud'homme. ©2005 Eurekah.com and Kluwer Academic / Plenum Publishers.

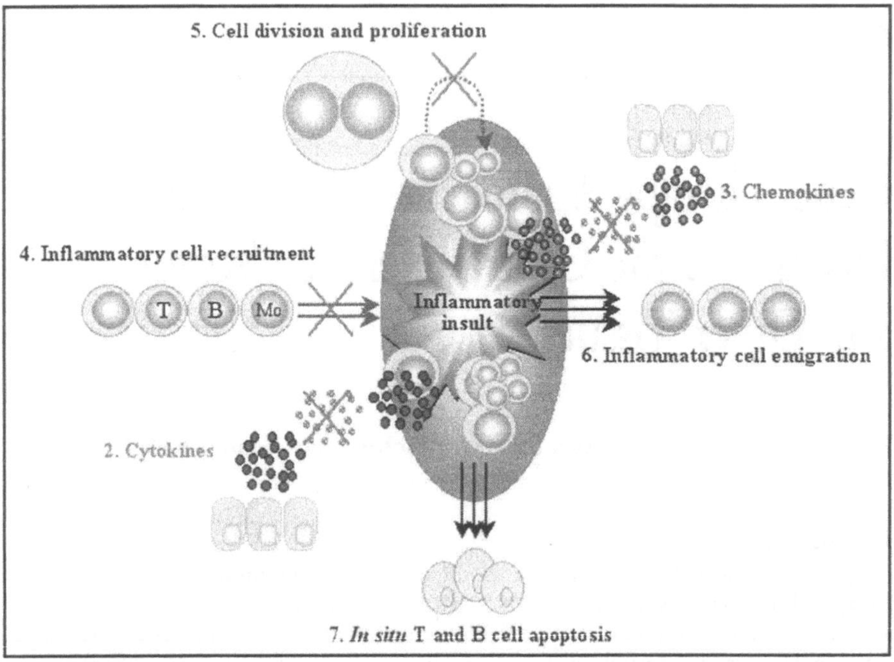

Figure 1. Targets for gene therapy intervention in autoimmunity. Most gene therapy approaches developed so far for autoimmune disorders are aimed at interfering with the different mechanisms and/or molecules sustaining the immune-mediated inflammatory processes responsible for the autoimmune insult. Thus, many attempts have been designed for delivering into the target organ heterologous genes coding for anti-inflammatory cytokines and chemokines[2,3] or for molecules able to down-regulate the production of pro-inflammatory cytokines and chemokines.[2,3] Gene therapy approaches aim to block co-stimulation or to antagonize antigen-specific T cell responses may interfere with the recruitment of inflammatory cells [T cells, B cells, monocytes/macrophages (Mo)] within the target organ.[4] These latter gene therapy strategies can be also used to in situ inhibit inflammatory cell division and proliferation.[5] Finally, several gene therapy protocols have been developed to foster inflammatory cells emigration from the target organ[6] or to induce in situ apopotosis of T and B cells.[7]

Different gene therapy strategies have been developed in the last ten years. The majority of these strategies aim at interfering with the immune-mediated inflammatory mechanisms sustaining and regulating autoimmune events (Fig. 1). Among them, the most interesting ones include: (i) inhibition of pro-inflammatory cytokines or chemokines; (ii) fostering immune deviation towards a protective Th2 profile; (iii) modulation of co-stimulation, (iv) induction of apoptosis of inflammatory cells; and, (v) induction of antigen-specific tolerance. Furthermore, in the most recent years, gene therapy of autoimmunity has been developed to replace crucial molecules destroyed by the autoimmune attack or, more in general, to replace the damaged tissue (e.g., microangiopathy, neuropathy, or wound healing in diabetes). These different gene therapy approaches have been so far mainly tested in animal models of MS, IDDM and RA. Our review will focus on these disorders.

Gene Therapy Tools

Apart form the selection of the right molecules to deliver within autoimmune tissues, a critical issue in gene therapy of autoimmunity is the selection of the appropriate tool for gene transfer purposes. Three main methodologies have been established. (i) The first one aims at the systemic release of the therapeutic molecules by delivering into muscles, liver, or blood stream the therapeutic genes engineered into viral vectors, liposomes or naked DNA. (ii) The second approach, which has received much attention from the scientific community, is based on the use of antigen-specific T or B cells (engineered mainly with retroviral vectors) as Trojan horses to deliver therapeutic molecule within autoimmune tissues. Antigen-specific T or B cells home "physiologically" into tissues where they can encounter the target antigen, which is usually confined within the autoimmune tissue. (iii) The third approach is mainly based on the transfer of the genes coding for the therapeutic molecules directly into the autoimmune tissues [e.g., central nervous system (CNS)] in order to provide a local therapy, which, in principle, should be more efficient. All three different approaches will be discussed although a detailed specification of the molecular characteristics of the biological and non biological vectors used to transfer heterologous gene within autoimmune tissue is beyond the scope of this chapter.

Cytokines, Chemokines and Cytokine Receptors

Cytokines, chemokines and their receptors are, by far, the most frequently used molecules in gene therapy of experimental autoimmunity since they represent plausible gene therapy targets (Table 1). This is due to the general understanding of the basic immunological mechanisms sustaining the pathogenesis of autoimmune disorders. The Th1 arm (e.g., Th1 $CD4^+$ cells and Th1 cytokines) of the adaptive immunity is thought to sustain cell-mediated autoimmune processes and macrophage-mediated pathologies via the secretion of pro-inflammatory cytokines and chemokines [e.g., interferon (IFN)γ and interleukin (IL)-12, and chemokines, such as RANTES, macrophage inflammatory protein (MIP)-1α and MIP-1β] showing disease-promoting activity. This detrimental pathway is usually counter-balanced by Th2-mediated immune responses,[4,5] which are sustained by Th2 cytokines–e.g., IL-4 IL-10, and IL-13–mainly acting as inhibitory molecules. Furthermore, the Th1 arm of the immune response is also induced and sustained by primary inflammatory cytokines [e.g., IL 1β, tumour necrosis factor (TNF)α, and IL-6].

Interleukin-4

The most widely used cytokine for the gene therapy of autoimmunity has been IL-4, the prototypical Th2 cytokine.

IL-4 has been administered systemically to EAE mice—either into the blood stream[8] or into resting or proliferating muscle cells[6]—without any substantial therapeutic effect. On the other hand, amelioration of EAE was obtained when the IL-4 gene was delivered directly into the CNS or through myelin-specific T cells.[22] Direct CNS injection in EAE has been accomplished by complexing the IL-4 gene with lipofectin[6] or by engineering the gene into partially replicating or non-replicating herpes simplex virus type-1 (HSV-1)-derived vectors.[21] While lipofectin-complexed IL-4 gene has been injected into the CNS parenchyma, these HSV-1 vectors have been injected into the cerebrospinal fluid (CSF),[24] the so-called ependymal route.[139] This latter approach showed to be feasible, safe, and therapeutically efficacious not only in mice but also in non-human primates with EAE.[24]

The IL-4 gene has been therapeutically used also in the animal model of RA, namely collagen-induced arthritis (CIA). Disease amelioration was obtained either by the intra-joint delivery of the IL-4 gene,[25-28] by intra-muscular adeno-associated virus (AAV)-mediated delivery,[29] or by using IL-4 gene-transfected dendritic cells or T cells.[30-31,35] Xenogeneic cells engineered to release IL-4 and placed intraperitoneally in biocompatible permeable capsules have been also effective in ameliorating CIA.[32-34]

Table 1. Genes and vectors for the therapy of autoimmune diseases

Therapeutic[a] Gene	Experimental Disease	Delivery Route	Gene Vector	Refs.
Cytokines—Chemokines				
IFNβ	EAE/MS	Local	Liposomes	6
	RA	Systemic	Retrovirus	7
IFNγ	EAE/MS	Local, systemic	Vaccinia virus, HSV-1	8,9
IL-1β	EAE/MS	Systemic	Vaccinia virus	8
IL-1ra	EAE/MS	Local	HSV-1	R.F., unpublished
	RA	Local	HSV-1, Retrovirus, Adenovirus	10-16
IL-2	EAE/MS	Systemic	Vaccinia virus	8
IL-4	EAE/MS	Local, systemic, T cells	Retrovirus, HSV-1, Vaccinia virus, Liposomes, Naked DNA	6,8,17-24
	RA	Local, systemic, T cells	Adenovirus, Retrovirus, AAV, Plasmid	25-35
	IDDM	Systemic, T cells	Retrovirus, AAV, Plasmid, Polymers	36-41
IL-6	EAE/MS	Systemic	Vaccinia virus	8
IL-10	EAE/MS	Local, systemic, T cells	Retrovirus, Vaccinia virus, Adenovirus, Liposomes, HSV-1	6,8,17-18,21,42-44
	RA	Local, systemic, T cells	Adenovirus, Plasmid, Naked DNA	45-48
	IDDM	Systemic, T cells	Retrovirus, AAV, Plasmid	38-39,49-50
Viral IL-10	RA	Local, systemic	Adenovirus	51-55
	IDDM	Systemic	AAV	56
IL12p40	RA	T cells	Retrovirus	57
	IDDM	Systemic	Adenovirus	58
IL-13	RA	Systemic	Plasmid	32-34
IP-10	EAE/MS	Systemic	Naked DNA	59
IKKβ	RA	Local	Adenovirus	60
TGF-β	EAE/MS	Systemic, local, T cells	Retrovirus, Liposomes, Naked DNA	6,19,61
	RA	Systemic, T cells	Retrovirus, Plasmid	62-63
	IDDM	Systemic	Plasmid	64
Cytokine receptors				
IL-1RII	RA	Local	Plasmid	65-66
IFNγR	IDDM	Systemic	Plasmid	39,67
TNFR-Ig	EAE/MS	Local, systemic	Liposomes	6
	RA	Local, systemic	Adenovirus	67-70
STNFR	EAE/MS	Local, systemic	Liposomes, Retrovirus	6,71
	RA	Local, T cells	AAV, Retrovirus	72-73
Apoptosis—Cell death				
CTLA4-IgG	EAE/MS	Systemic	Adenovirus	74
	RA	Local	Adenovirus	75
FasL	EAE/MS	Systemic	Naked DNA	76
	RA	Local, T cells	Adenovirus, Plasmid	77-78
Bcl-2	IDDM	Local	Adenovirus	769
P16INK4a	RA	Local	Adenovirus	80-81
p21CIP1	RA	Local	Adenovirus	81
Thymidine kinase	RA	Local	Adenovirus	82

continued on next page

Table 1. Continued

Therapeutic[a] Gene	Experimental Disease	Delivery Route	Gene Vector	Refs.
Antigens				
PLP	EAE/MS	Systemic, B cells	Retrovirus, Naked DNA	20,83
MOG	EAE/MS	Systemic	Naked DNA	20
MBP-IgG1	EAE/MS	B cells	Retrovirus	84
GAD	IDDM	Systemic, B cells	Vaccinia, Plasmid	85-87
Growth factors—Tissue repair molecules				
EFG	IDDM	Local	AAV	88
VEGF	IDDM	Systemic, local	Adenovirus, Plasmid, Liposomes	89-92
PDGFα	EAE/MS	T cells	Retrovirus	93
FGF-I	IDDM	Local	Naked DNA	94
FGF-II	EAE/MS	Local	HSV-1	95
IGF-I	IDDM	Local	Adenovirus	96
Insulin	IDDM	Systemic	Adenovirus, Retrovirus, AAV, Liposomes, Plasmid	97-122
NGF	EAE/MS	T cells	Retrovirus	123
	IDDM	Local	HSV-1	124-125
NT-3	IDDM	Systemic	Adenovirus	126
PDX-1	IDDM	Local	Adenovirus	127
NeuroD				
betacellulin	IDDM	Local	Adenovirus	128
Adrenomedullin	IDDM	Systemic	Adenovirus	129
Glucokinase	IDDM	Systemic	Adenovirus	130
Kallikrein	IDDM	Local	Plasmid	131
GKRP	IDDM	Systemic	Adenovirus	132
ORP150	IDDM	Systemic	Adenovirus	133
IRS-1	IDDM	Systemic	Adenovirus	134
iNOS	IDDM	Local	Adenovirus	135
Leptin	IDDM	Systemic	Adenovirus, AAV	136-137
TIMP-1, TIMP-3	RA	Local	Adenovirus	138

[a]Abbreviations: IFN = interferon; IL = interleukin; IL-1ra = IL-1 receptor antagonist; IKKβ = inhibitor of neuclear factor Kβ; TGF = transforming growth factor; IL-1R = IL-1 receptor; IFNγR = IFNγ receptor; TNF = tumor necrosis factor; TNFR-Ig; TNF receptor-Ig fusion protein; sTNFR = soluble TNF receptor; CTLA = Cytotoxic T Lymphocyte Antigen; FasL = Fas ligand; PLP = proteolipid protein; MOG = myelin oligodendrocyte glycoprotein; MBP = myelin basic protein; GAD = glutamic acid decarboxylase; EGF = epidermal growth factor; VEGF = vascular endothelial growth factor; PDGF = platelet derived growth factor; FGF = fibroblast growth factor; IGF = insulin-like growth factor; NGF = nerve growth factor; NT = neurotrophin; GKRP = glucokinase regulatory protein; ORP = oxygen regulated protein; IRS = insulin receptor substrate; iNOS = inducible nitric oxide synthetase; TIMP = tissue inhibitors of metalloproteases.

In nonobese diabetic (NOD) mice, spontaneously developing IDDM, IL-4 gene therapy has been only partially successful. Intramuscular AAV-mediated administration of the IL-4 gene was ineffective[38] while intramuscular injection of a plasmid coding for an IL-4-Ig fusion protein ameliorated the experimental disease.[41] I.v. injection of IL-4-coding plasmids prevented diabetes only when used in combination with an IL-10-expressing plasmid.[39] On the other hand, experimental diabetes was ameliorated when the i.v. injected IL-4 plasmid was complexed in polymers.[37] Finally, antigen-specific T cells [glutamic acid decarboxylase (GAD-specific)]—engineered to constitutively release IL-4—efficiently prevented the onset of experimental diabetes.[36,40]

Interleukin-10

IL-10 has been also extensively used in gene therapy protocols of autoimmunity. I.v. injection of IL-10-expressing Vaccinia virus ameliorated EAE in mice.[8] Proteolipid protein (PLP)-specific T cells engineered with the IL-10 gene were therapeutically effective in PLP-induced EAE,[42] but not in myelin basic protein (MBP)-induced EAE.[17] Either fibroblasts transfected with the IL-10 gene and transplanted into the brain[44] or IL-10-expressing adenoviral vectors injected into the CSF through the ependymal route,[43] showed to be beneficial in EAE. By contrast, IL-10 was ineffective when injected into the brain parenchyma with liposomes,[18] adenoviruses,[28] or partially replicating HSV-1 vectors.[29]

Mouse IL-10, or the viral IL-10 (vIL-10) analogue produced by the Epstein-Barr virus, has been used in experimental models of RA. Intra-joint administration of vIL-10-expressing adenoviruses has been reported to inhibit experimental arthritis[51-53] but, at the same time, it also induced synovial inflammation.[54] T cells transfected with an IL-10-containing plasmid ameliorated RA in mice.[46] Positive results have been also obtained by

i. i.v. injection of IL-10 or vIL-10 expressing adenoviral vectors,[47,51,54]
ii. plasmid-mediated muscle transfer of IL-10,[48] and,
iii. intradermal injection of an IL-10 bearing plasmid.[45]

IL-10 gene therapy was shown to be effective also in experimental diabetes. I.v. injection of both AAV vectors expressing IL-10[38] or vIL-10[56] and plasmids containing the IL-10 and the IL-4 genes[39] efficiently prevented the onset of diabetes in NOD mice. The same results have been obtained when the IL-10 gene was transferred into islet-specific Th1 cells, which were, in turn, re-infused into diabetic mice.[50] Recurrence of autoimmune diabetes has also been prevented through pancreatic islet transplantation followed by i.v. administration of an IL-10-expressing AAV vector.[49]

Other Cytokines and Chemokines

Among gene therapy protocols aimed at interfering with pathogenic Th1 cells, those using the Th2 cytokine IL-13 have been very efficacious in ameliorating animal models of RA.[32-34]

Positive results in autoimmune models have been obtained by using soluble cytokine receptors acting as decoy molecules—i.e., IFNγ receptor (IFNγR) in diabetes[41,67]—or as receptor antagonists—i.e., IL-12p40 in RA[57] and diabetes.[58]

Vaccination with naked DNA against the chemokine IFNγ-inducible protein (IP)-10 was able to ameliorate EAE by redirecting antigen-specific T cell polarization.[59]

TGFβ, a cytokine known to have regulatory/suppressor functions on Th1 cells, has been used in EAE[6,19,61] as well as RA[62,63] and diabetes[64] but the results have been contradictory.

The local delivery of IFNβ in EAE[6] and RA[7] showed positive results. On the other hand, local, but not systemic, delivery of the prototypical Th1 cytokine IFNγ, has been shown to dramatically improve EAE.[9] This was mainly due to the ability of IFNγ to induce programmed cell death of pathogenic T cells infiltrating the CNS.[9]

Primary inflammatory cytokines–IL-1 and TNFα—have been also the target of several gene therapy studies. IL-1 receptor antagonist (IL-1ra) gene delivery within the CNS of EAE mice has been able to delay onset and decrease disease severity (R.F. personal communication). Intra-synovial delivery of IL-1ra—using HSV-1, retroviral, or adenoviral vectors—has been shown to be very effective in preventing joint inflammation and destruction.[10-16] Similar result has been obtained by the delivery of the IL-1 receptor II (IL-1RII) decoy receptor into RA mice.[65,66] Gene therapy approaches based on the use of soluble forms of the TNF receptors (TNFR) or of TNFR-Ig fusion proteins have been developed. In EAE, systemic delivery of TNF receptors was ineffective while local administration was efficacious in ameliorating the disease course.[6,71] Systemic, local, and T cell-mediated administration of genes coding for TNF receptors into RA mice, have shown to be very effective in the treatment of joint inflammation,[6,66-70,72-73] although a rebound to greater inflammatory activity in later time points has been also described.[68] Finally, the constitutive expression of IkappaB kinase (IKK)β—a modulator of the pro-inflammatory transcription factor NFkappaβ—obtained by intra-articular adenoviral-mediated gene delivery, has been shown to be an alternative, original and efficient anti-inflammatory gene therapy strategy in a rat model of RA.[60]

Molecules Modulating Apoptosis

An alternative strategy, fostering programmed cell death of both effector T cells and cells target of the autoimmune reaction, has been pursued in several gene therapy studies.

Local delivery of adenoviral vectors expressing the fusion protein cytotoxic T lymphocyte-associated protein (CTLA)Ig—a co-stimulatory molecule implicated in the apoptosis of activated T cells—has been therapeutically successful in EAE,[74] and RA.[75]

Fas ligand (FasL) gene delivery, obtained using DNA vaccination protocols, was shown to be able to elicit the generation of blocking anti-FasL antibodies. This approach had contradictory effects in EAE, being effective when administered at onset of the disease but detrimental when administered later on during the disease course.[76] Local delivery of FasL using adenoviral vectors or T cells was able to induce target cell death and amelioration of RA.[76-77] It is interesting to note that, the local induction of apoptosis in animal model of RA was effective not only in inducing apoptosis of auto aggressive T cells, but also in obtaining apoptosis of synoviocytes (therapeutic synovectomy). Similar results have been obtained when adenoviral vectors coding for genes involved in the cell cycle—such as P16INK4a[80-81] and p21CIP1[81]—were used in the mouse models of RA. The same results have been obtained by intra-articularly injection of adenoviral vectors coding for the suicide gene thymidine kinase to non-human primates,[82] an approach that will be soon tested also in humans.[140]

A different approach has been taken in diabetes. Anti-apoptotic Bcl-2 gene has been transferred to pancreatic islets before transplantation and a protective effect has been observed.[79]

Antigen-Based Therapy

A novel and interesting gene therapy approach has been recently proposed. Mice susceptible to autoimmune disorders have been transformed into resistant mice by down regulating auto reactive T-cells using different gene therapy strategies.

In EAE, B cells were genetically modified to constitutively express the SJL-specific PLP-encephalitogenic determinant (aa139-151) and then adoptively transferred into syngeneic hosts. This protocol induced PLP-specific unresponsiveness thus protecting the majority of mice (from 62% to 83%) from EAE induction. In the remaining mice, disease onset was delayed and disease severity was ameliorated.[83] In another study, a retroviral construct—expressing a chimeric IgG-MBP construct—was engineered into B cells and intravenously injected into syngenic EAE mice. B cells ameliorated ongoing EAE when passively transferred. The effect was specific and did not involve bystander suppression since MBP-IgG did not affect the disease course when induced by immunization with the PLP immunodominant peptide plus MBP.[84] It has also been shown that the co-delivery of the IL-4 gene with a DNA vaccine encoding the self-peptide PLP139-151 or with the myelin oligodendrocyte glycoprotein (MOG) gene, protected mice from EAE.[20]

Similar results have obtained in experimental models of diabetes. B cells engineered to release a GAD-Ig fusion protein prevented autoimmune insulitis in NOD mice.[86] Systemic injection of a Vaccinia virus-derived vector coding for GAD was also able to prevent autoimmune diabetes.[85] Finally, vaccination with a plasmid DNA encoding for GAD protected from autoimmune diabetes; however, disease susceptibility was restored when B7/CD28 co-stimulation was provided.[87]

Tissue Repair and Replacement

The gene therapy approaches, described so far, have been attempted in order to prevent tissue damage. However, organ-specific autoimmune diseases become clinically evident when anatomical and functional tissue damage is already established. It is then imperative to look for new tools (i) to revert the tissue damage, (ii) to replace the non-functioning organ or (iii) to foster endogenous repairing mechanisms. Gene therapy has been used to prove the therapeutic efficacy of these novel approaches.

Autoimmune Diabetes

Insulin Replacement

Gene therapy-mediated strategies aimed to replace non-functioning organs are possible in a disease like autoimmune diabetes where a single, metabolically crucial, molecule—such as insulin—can be used to replace non-functioning pancreatic islets. The transfer of the insulin gene to revert autoimmune diabetes has been the most common gene therapy approach so far used.[97-122] Insulin gene therapy has, however, at least three major drawbacks which have to be taken into consideration: (i) insulin is a heterodimeric protein originating from the specific cleavage of the precursor protein pro-insulin in β-cells; (ii) insulin release needs tight regulation since excessive production leads to hypoglycaemic coma and death; and, (iii) insulin has to be released into the blood stream to reach the whole body. To solve, at least partially, these problems, several groups have attempted to transfer the pro-insulin gene[100,122]—which is active at lower levels compared to the mature insulin. Most of the studies have been based on the modification of the insulin cleavage site in order to render the modified pro-insulin sensitive to furin-mediated proteolysis.[97,99] Alternatively, diabetes was reverted in NOD mice by the gene transfer of a single chain insulin analogue, which leads to the production of a biologically active molecule.[109] Regulation of insulin transgene expression has been also the matter of intense investigations. These studies have yielded contradictory results. The use of the native insulin promoter in hepatocytes has failed.[101] The G6pase promoter has been successfully employed in hepatocytes.[107-108] Synthetic promoters with glucose sensitive elements or insulin sensitive inhibiting elements have been shown to determine a certain degree of regulation in insulin release.[97-110] A promoter under the control of an exogenously administered drug (rapamycin) has been also proposed.[101] The most different combinations of gene delivery tools have been also attempted to obtain systemic release of insulin. Naked plasmid DNA, or liposomes, coding for insulin have been transferred to muscle,[99,102,106,110,113] to hepatocytes[97] or engineered into transplanted fibroblasts[122] or exocrine glands.[118] Procedures aimed to deliver such constructs into the blood stream have been also attempted.[111,119] Since adenoviral vectors display a high tropism for hepatocytes after i.v. administration, adenoviral-mediated insulin gene delivery has been the mostly used.[98,101-102,107-109,112] However, several other tissues such as liver,[103] adipose tissue,[104] and pancreas,[105] have been proposed as an alternative target. Insulin gene-containing adeno-associated viral vectors have been injected into muscles,[100,116] into haematopoietic cells,[115] and into the liver.[117] Retroviruses have been used to insert the insulin gene into fibroblasts[114] and hepatocytes[120] before transplantation.

Other Approaches (Developmental and Growth Factors)

An alternative and original approach aimed to tissue replacement by gene therapy has been also recently proposed in autoimmune diabetes. The gene transfer of developmental factors (e.g., PDX-1; combination of neuroD and betacellulin) able to induce the neogenesis of pancreatic islets in the liver has been established using adenoviral-mediated gene transfer.[127-128] Gene therapy protocols employing growth or angiogenic factors have been used in experimental diabetes. The goal was to prevent secondary damages thus possibly increasing wound healing. Several of these attempts are reported in Table 1. Among the most promising gene therapy approaches, those employing vascular endothelial growth factor (VEGF) and epidermal growth factor (EGF) genes have been already successfully tested in pre-clinical studies.[88-92] Many other molecules are under scrutiny.[97,124-137] It is noteworthy that a human trial based on local delivery of the VEGF gene in diabetic patients is currently ongoing.[141]

EAE Studies

Growth Factors

Fostering the tissue endogenous repair mechanisms thus replacing non-functioning myelin forming cells has been the matter of several studies in EAE. So far, only neurothrophic growth factor gene therapy has been attempted to reach the goal. Encephalitogenic mouse T cells transfected with an antigen-inducible transgene for platelet-derived growth factor (PDGF)α—a growth factor important in regulating the development of oligodendrocytes—migrated into the CNS where they released PDGFα that, in turn, ameliorated ongoing EAE.[93] MBP-specific $CD4^+$ T cells transduced with a recombinant retrovirus encoding nerve growth factor (NGF) have been also used in EAE. These modified T cells efficiently suppressed clinical EAE induced by non-transduced MBP-specific T cells, possibly also interfering with the inflammatory cascade.[123] Injection through the ependymal route of HSV-1-derived vectors coding for fibroblast growth factor (FGF)-II—a growth factor inducing differentiation and proliferation of oligodendrocyte progenitors—was shown to be able to ameliorate ongoing EAE without toxic reaction.[95] However, EAE was ameliorated when FGF-II gene therapy was administered for up to 4 weeks but not when it was administered for longer periods of time (i.e., months) since chronic FGF-II administration induced diffuse astrocytic proliferation thus blocking terminal differentiation of oligodendrocyte progenitors.

Conclusions

The gene therapy of autoimmunity has held many promises for the last ten years, owing to its potential as an alternative therapeutic approach for diseases lacking a definitive cure and with a devastating social impact. However, there are still several issues to solve before these approaches would be transferable to humans.

Some studies are conceptually non applicable to human diseases. For instance, T and B cell-based antigen-specific approaches are difficult to translate into the clinical practice since the pathogenic (auto)antigens in MS, RA, and IDDM are not yet completely identified and antigen heterogeneity occurs in patients during the course of the disease. From a technological point of view, many gene transfer tools cannot be used in humans due to their (i) toxicity or immunogenicity (i.e., Vaccinia virus, HSV-1, first generation adenoviral vectors), (ii) scarce gene transfer efficiency (i.e., naked DNA, liposomes), and (iii) short-term expression (Vaccinia, HSV-1, naked DNA, liposomes).

However, the huge amounts of data generated in the last decade in experimental models have been very instrumental to weight the potential detrimental vs. protective effect of this novel therapeutic approach. We know for example that it is much more safer and efficacious to transfer the "therapeutic" gene directly into the autoimmune target organ rather than into the systemic circulation. This approach has several advantages: (i) restricted area (i.e., the CSF and the synovia) to target thus more efficient gene transfer, (ii) higher levels of transgene expression in the damaged/target area; and, (iii) no peripheral side/toxic effects.

In conclusion, while gene therapy approaches of autoimmune diseases are promising, there is a long way ahead before envisaging a wide application of this new technology in human diseases. While gene therapy approaches aimed to recovery loss of functions have shown in experimental models of autoimmunity great efficacy and reproducibility, without over toxic effect, there is still a lot to do for gene therapy protocols aimed to replace non-functioning organs.

Acknowledgments

Our work is supported by Minister of Health (Progetti Finalizzati), Minister of University and Research (MIUR) and Italian National Multiple Sclerosis Society (AISM).

References

1. Evans CH, Robbins PD, Ghivizzani SC et al. Clinical trial to assess the safety, feasibility, and efficacy of transferring a potentially anti-arthritic cytokine gene to human joints with rheumatoid arthritis. Hum Gene Ther 1996; 7:1261-1280.
2. Kay MA, Glorioso JC, Naldini L. Viral vectors for gene therapy: the art of turning infectious agents into vehicles of therapeutics. Nat Med 2001; 7:33-40.
3. Martino G, Poliani PL, Marconi PC et al. Cytokine gene therapy of autoimmune demyelination revisited using herpes simplex virus type-1-derived vectors. Gene Ther 2000; 7:1087-1093.
4. Abbas AK, Murphy KM, Sher A. Functional diversity of helper T lymphocytes. Nature 1996; 383:787-793.
5. Adorini L. Cytokine-based immunointervention in the treatment of autoimmune diseases. Clin Exp Immunol 2003; 132:185-192.
6. Croxford JL, Triantaphyllopoulos K, Podhajcer OL et al. Cytokine gene therapy in experimental allergic encephalomyelitis by injection of plasmid DNA-cationic liposome complex into the central nervous system. J Immunol 1998; 160:5181-5187.
7. Triantaphyllopoulos KA, Williams RO, Tailor H et al. Amelioration of collagen-induced arthritis and suppression of interferon-gamma, interleukin-12, and tumor necrosis factor alpha production by interferon-beta gene therapy. Arthritis Rheum 1999; 42:90-99.
8. Willenborg DO, Fordham SA, Cowden WB et al. Cytokines and murine autoimmune encephalomyelitis: inhibition or enhancement of disease with antibodies to select cytokines, or by delivery of exogenous cytokines using a recombinant vaccinia virus system. Scand J Immunol 1995; 41:31-40.
9. Furlan R, Brambilla E, Ruffini F et al. Intrathecal delivery of IFN-gamma protects C57BL/6 mice from chronic-progressive experimental autoimmune encephalomyelitis by increasing apoptosis of central nervous system-infiltrating lymphocytes. J Immunol 2001; 167:1821-1829.
10. Otani K, Nita I, Macaulay W et al. Suppression of antigen-induced arthritis in rabbits by ex vivo gene therapy. J Immunol 1996; 156:3558-3562.
11. Oligino T, Ghivizzani S, Wolfe D et al. Intra-articular delivery of a herpes simplex virus IL-1Ra gene vector reduces inflammation in a rabbit model of arthritis. Gene Ther 1999; 6:1713-1720.
12. Hung GL, Galea-Lauri J, Mueller GM et al. Suppression of intra-articular responses to interleukin-1 by transfer of the interleukin-1 receptor antagonist gene to synovium. Gene Ther 1994; 1:64-69.
13. Makarov SS, Olsen JC, Johnston WN et al. Suppression of experimental arthritis by gene transfer of interleukin 1 receptor antagonist cDNA. Proc Natl Acad Sci USA 1996; 93:402-406.
14. Bandara G, Mueller GM, Galea-Lauri J et al. Intraarticular expression of biologically active interleukin 1-receptor-antagonist protein by ex vivo gene transfer. Proc Natl Acad Sci USA 1993; 90:10764-10768.
15. Bakker AC, Joosten LA, Arntz OJ et al. Prevention of murine collagen-induced arthritis in the knee and ipsilateral paw by local expression of human interleukin-1 receptor antagonist protein in the knee. Arthritis Rheum 1997; 40:893-900.
16. Roessler BJ, Hartman JW, Vallance DK et al. Inhibition of interleukin-1-induced effects in synoviocytes transduced with the human IL-1 receptor antagonist cDNA using an adenoviral vector. Hum Gene Ther 1995; 6:307-316.
17. Martino G, Poliani PL, Marconi PC et al. Cytokine gene therapy of autoimmune demyelination revisited using herpes simplex virus type-1-derived vectors. Gene Ther 2000; 7:1087-1093.
18. Shaw MK, Lorens JB, Dhawan A et al. Local delivery of interleukin 4 by retrovirus-transduced T lymphocytes ameliorates experimental autoimmune encephalomyelitis. J Exp Med 1997; 185:1711-1714.
19. Piccirillo CA, Prud'homme GJ. Prevention of experimental allergic encephalomyelitis by intramuscular gene transfer with cytokine-encoding plasmid vectors. Hum Gene Ther 1999; 10:1915-1922.

20. Garren H, Ruiz PJ, Watkins TA et al. Combination of gene delivery and DNA vaccination to protect from and reverse Th1 autoimmune disease via deviation to the Th2 pathway. Immunity 2001; 15:15-22.
21. Broberg E, Setala N, Roytta M et al. Expression of interleukin-4 but not of interleukin-10 from a replicative herpes simplex virus type 1 viral vector precludes experimental allergic encephalomyelitis Gene Ther 2001; 8:769-777.
22. Furlan R, Poliani PL, Galbiati F et al. Central nervous system delivery of interleukin-4 by a non-replicative herpes simplex type 1 viral vector ameliorates autoimmune demyelination. Hum Gene Ther 1998; 9:2605-2617.
23. Furlan R, Poliani PL, Marconi PC et al. Central nervous system gene therapy with interleukin-4 inhibits progression of ongoing relapsing-remitting autoimmune encephalomyelitis in Biozzi AB/H mice. Gene Ther 2001; 8:13-19.
24. Poliani PL, Brok H, Furlan R et al. Delivery to the central nervous system of a nonreplicative herpes simplex type 1 vector engineered with the interleukin 4 gene protects rhesus monkeys from hyperacute autoimmune encephalomyelitis. Hum Gene Ther 2001; 12:905-920.
25. Lubberts E, Joosten LA, van Den Bersselaar L et al. Adenoviral vector-mediated overexpression of IL-4 in the knee joint of mice with collagen-induced arthritis prevents cartilage destruction. J Immunol 1999; 163:4546-4556.
26. Woods JM, Katschke KJ, Volin MV et al. IL-4 adenoviral gene therapy reduces inflammation, proinflammatory cytokines, vascularization, and bony destruction in rat adjuvant-induced arthritis. J Immunol 2001; 166:1214-1222.
27. Lubberts E, Joosten LA, Chabaud M et al. IL-4 gene therapy for collagen arthritis suppresses synovial IL-17 and osteoprotegerin ligand and prevents bone erosion. J Clin Invest 2000; 105:1697-1710.
28. Boyle DL, Nguyen KH, Zhuang S, Intra-articular IL-4 gene therapy in arthritis: anti-inflammatory effect and enhanced th2activity. Gene Ther 1999; 6:1911-1918.
29. Cottard V, Mulleman D, Bouille P et al. Adeno-associated virus-mediated delivery of IL-4 prevents collagen-induced arthritis. Gene Ther 2000; 7:1930-1939.
30. Morita Y, Yang J, Gupta R et al. Dendritic cells genetically engineered to express IL-4 inhibit murine collagen-induced arthritis. J Clin Invest 2001; 107:1275-1284.
31. Kim SH, Kim S, Evans CH et al. Effective treatment of established murine collagen-induced ar thritis by systemic administration of dendritic cells genetically modified to express IL-4. J Immunol 2001; 166:3499-3505.
32. Bessis N, Honiger J, Damotte D et al. Encapsulation in hollow fibres of xenogeneic cells engineered to secrete IL-4 or IL-13 ameliorates murine collagen-induced arthritis (CIA). Clin Exp Immunol 1999; 117:376-382.
33. Bessis N, Chiocchia G, Kollias G et al. Modulation of proinflammatory cytokine production in tumour necrosis factor-alpha (TNF-alpha)-transgenic mice by treatment with cells engineered to secrete IL-4, IL-10 or IL-13. Clin Exp Immunol 1998; 111:391-396.
34. Bessis N, Boissier MC, Ferrara P et al. Attenuation of collagen-induced arthritis in mice by treatment with vector cells engineered to secrete interleukin-13. Eur J Immunol 1996; 26:2399-2403.
35. Tarner IH, Nakajima A, Seroogy CM et al. Retroviral gene therapy of collagen-induced arthritis by local delivery of IL-4. Clin Immunol 2002; 105:304-314.
36. Zipris D, Karnieli E. A single treatment with IL-4 via retrovirally transduced lymphocytes partially protects against diabetes in BioBreeding (BB) rats. JOP 2002; 3:76-82.
37. Lee M, Koh JJ, Han SO et al. Prevention of autoimmune insulitis by delivery of interleukin-4 plasmid using a soluble and biodegradable polymeric carrier. Pharm Res 2002; 19:246-249.
38. Goudy K, Song S, Wasserfall C et al. Adeno-associated virus vector-mediated IL-10 gene delivery prevents type 1 diabetes in NOD mice. Proc Natl Acad Sci USA 2001; 98:13913-13918.
39. Ko KS, Lee M, Koh JJ et al. Combined administration of plasmids encoding IL-4 and IL-10 prevents the development of autoimmune diabetes in nonobese diabetic mice. Mol Ther 2001; 4:313-316.

40. Yamamoto AM, Chernajovsky Y, Lepault F et al. The activity of immunoregulatory T cells mediating active tolerance is potentiated in nonobese diabetic mice by an IL-4-based retroviral gene therapy. J Immunol 2001; 166:4973-4980.
41. Chang Y, Prud'homme GJ. Intramuscular administration of expression plasmids encoding interferon-gamma receptor/IgG1 or IL-4/IgG1 chimeric proteins protects from autoimmunity. J Gene Med 1999;1:415-423.
42. Mathisen PM, Yu M, Johnson JM et al. Treatment of experimental autoimmune encephalomyelitis with genetically modified memory T cells. J Exp Med 1997; 186:159-164.
43. Cua DJ, Hutchins B, LaFace DM et al. Central nervous system expression of IL-10 inhibits autoimmune encephalomyelitis. J Immunol 2001; 166:602-608.
44. Croxford JL, Feldmann M, Chernajovsky Y et al. Different therapeutic outcomes in experimental allergic encephalomyelitis dependant upon the mode of delivery of IL-10: a comparison of the effects of protein, adenoviral or retroviral IL-10 delivery into the central nervous system. J Immunol 2001; 166:4124-4130.
45. Miyata M, Sasajima T, Sato H et al. Suppression of collagen induced arthritis in mice utilizing plasmid DNA encoding interleukin 10. J Rheumatol 2000; 27:1601-1605.
46. Setoguchi K, Misaki Y, Araki Y et al. Antigen-specific T cells transduced with IL-10 ameliorate experimentally induced arthritis without impairing the systemic immune response to the antigen. J Immunol 2000; 165:5980-5986.
47. Quattrocchi E, Dallman MJ, Dhillon AP et al. Murine IL-10 gene transfer inhibits established collagen-induced arthritis and reduces adenovirus-mediated inflammatory responses in mouse liver. J Immunol 2001; 166:5970-5978.
48. Saidenberg-Kermanac'h N, Bessis N, Deleuze V et al. Efficacy of interleukin-10 gene electrotransfer into skeletal muscle in mice with collagen-induced arthritis. J Gene Med 2003; 5:164-171.
49. Zhang YC, Pileggi A, Agarwal A et al. Abstract Adeno-associated virus-mediated IL-10 gene therapy inhibits diabetes recurrence in syngeneic islet cell transplantation of NOD mice. Diabetes 2003; 52:708-716.
50. Moritani M, Yoshimoto K, Ii S et al. Prevention of adoptively transferred diabetes in nonobese diabetic mice with IL-10-transduced islet-specific Th1 lymphocytes. A gene therapy model for autoimmune diabetes. J Clin Invest 1996 15; 98:1851-1859.
51. Apparailly F, Verwaerde C, Jacquet C et al. Adenovirus-mediated transfer of viral IL-10 gene inhibits murine collagen-induced arthritis. J Immunol 1998; 160:5213-5220.
52. Whalen JD, Lechman EL, Carlos CA et al. Adenoviral transfer of the viral IL-10 gene periarticularly to mouse paws suppresses development of collagen-induced arthritis in both injected and uninjected paws. J Immunol 1999; 162:3625-3632.
53. Lechman ER, Jaffurs D, Ghivizzani SC et al. Direct adenoviral gene transfer of viral IL-10 to rabbit knees with experimental arthritis ameliorates disease in both injected and contralateral control knees. J Immunol 1999; 163:2202-2208.
54. Ma Y, Thornton S, Duwel LE et al. Inhibition of collagen-induced arthritis in mice by viral IL-10 gene transfer. J Immunol 1998; 161:1516-1524.
55. Kim SH, Evans CH, Kim S et al. Gene therapy for established murine collagen-induced arthritis by local and systemic adenovirus-mediated delivery of interleukin-4. Arthritis Res 2000; 2:293-302.
56. Yang Z, Chen M, Wu R et al. Suppression of autoimmune diabetes by viral IL-10 gene transfer. J Immunol 2002; 168:6479-6485.
57. Nakajima A, Seroogy CM, Sandora MR et al. Antigen-specific T cell-mediated gene therapy in collagen-induced arthritis. J Clin Invest 2001; 107:1293-1301.
58. Yasuda H, Nagata M, Arisawa K et al. Local expression of immunoregulatory IL-12p40 gene prolonged syngeneic islet graft survival in diabetic NOD mice. J Clin Invest 1998; 102:1807-1814.
59. Wildbaum G, Netzer N, Karin N. Plasmid DNA encoding IFN-gamma-inducible protein 10 redirects antigen-specific T cell polarization and suppresses experimental autoimmune encephalomyelitis. J Immunol 2002; 168:5885-5892.
60. Tak PP, Gerlag DM, Aupperle KR et al. Abstract Inhibitor of nuclear factor kappaB kinase beta is a key regulator of synovial inflammation. Arthritis Rheum 2001; 44:1897-1907.

61. Chen LZ, Hochwald GM, Huang C et al. Gene therapy in allergic encephalomyelitis using myelin basic protein-specific T cells engineered to express latent transforming growth factor-beta1. Proc Natl Acad Sci USA 1998; 95:12516-12521.
62. Song XY, Gu M, Jin WW et al. Plasmid DNA encoding transforming growth factor-beta1 suppresses chronic disease in a streptococcal cell wall-induced arthritis model. J Clin Invest 1998; 101:2615-2621.
63. Chernajovsky Y, Adams G, Triantaphyllopoulos K et al. Pathogenic lymphoid cells engineered to express TGF beta 1 ameliorate disease in a collagen-induced arthritis model. Gene Ther 1997; 4:553-559.
64. Piccirillo CA, Chang Y, Prud'homme GJ. TGF-beta1 somatic gene therapy prevents autoimmune disease in nonobese diabetic mice. J Immunol 1998; 161:3950-3956.
65. Bessis N, Guery L, Mantovani A et al. The type II decoy receptor of IL-1 inhibits murine collagen-induced arthritis. Eur J Immunol 2000; 30:867-875.
66. Ghivizzani SC, Lechman ER, Kang R et al. Direct adenovirus-mediated gene transfer of interleukin 1 and tumor necrosis factor alpha soluble receptors to rabbit knees with experimental arthritis has local and distal anti-arthritic effects. Proc Natl Acad Sci USA 1998; 95:4613-4618.
67. Prud'homme GJ, Chang Y. et al. Prevention of autoimmune diabetes by intramuscular gene therapy with a nonviral vector encoding an interferon-gamma receptor/IgG1 fusion protein. Gene Ther 1999; 6:771-777.
68. Quattrocchi E, Walmsley M, Browne K et al. Paradoxical effects of adenovirus-mediated blockade of TNF activity in murine collagen-induced arthritis. J Immunol 1999; 163:1000-1009.
69. Kolls J, Peppel K, Silva M et al. Prolonged and effective blockade of tumor necrosis factor activity through adenovirus-mediated gene transfer. Proc Natl Acad Sci USA 1994; 91:215-219.
70. Le CH, Nicolson AG, Morales A et al. Suppression of collagen-induced arthritis through adenovirus-mediated transfer of a modified tumor necrosis factor alpha receptor gene. Arthritis Rheum 1997; 40:1662-1669.
71. Croxford JL, Triantaphyllopoulos KA, Neve RM et al. Gene therapy for chronic relapsing experimental allergic encephalomyelitis using cells expressing a novel soluble p75 dimeric TNF receptor. J Immunol 2000; 164:2776-2781.
72. Zhang HG, Xie J, Yang P et al. Adeno-associated virus production of soluble tumor necrosis factor receptor neutralizes tumor necrosis factor alpha and reduces arthritis. Hum Gene Ther 2000; 11:2431-2442.
73. Chernajovsky Y, Adams G, Podhajcer OL et al. Inhibition of transfer of collagen-induced arthritis into SCID mice by ex vivo infection of spleen cells with retroviruses expressing soluble tumor necrosis factor receptor. Gene Ther 1995; 2:731-735.
74. Kawaguchi Y. A gene therapy or purified CTLA4IgG treatment of experimental allergic encephalomyelitis. Hokkaido Igaku Zasshi 1999; 74:467-475.
75. Ijima K, Murakami M, Okamoto H et al. Successful gene therapy via intraarticular injection of adenovirus vector containing CTLA4IgG in a murine model of type II collagen-induced arthritis. Hum Gene Ther 2001; 12:1063-1077.
76. Wildbaum G, Westermann J, Maor G et al. A targeted DNA vaccine encoding Fas ligand defines its dual role in the regulation of experimental autoimmune encephalomyelitis. J Clin Invest 2000; 106:671–679.
77. Zhang H, Yang Y, Horton JL et al. Amelioration of collagen-induced arthritis by CD95 (Apo-1/Fas)-ligand gene transfer. J Clin Invest 1997; 100:1951-1957.
78. Okamoto K, Asahara H, Kobayashi T et al. Induction of apoptosis in the rheumatoid synovium by Fas ligand gene transfer. Gene Ther 1998; 5:331-338.
79. Contreras JL, Bilbao G, Smyth CA et al. Cytoprotection of pancreatic islets before and early after transplantation using gene therapy. Kidney Int Suppl 2002; 61S1:79-84.
80. Nasu K, Kohsaka H, Nonomura Y et al. Adenoviral transfer of cyclin-dependent kinase inhibitor genes suppresses collagen-induced arthritis in mice. J Immunol 2000; 165:7246-7252.
81. Taniguchi K, Kohsaka H, Inoue N et al. Induction of the p16INK4a senescence gene as a new therapeutic strategy for the treatment of rheumatoid arthritis. Nat Med 1999; 5:760-767.

82. Goossens PH, Schouten GJ, 't Hart BA et al. Feasibility of adenovirus-mediated nonsurgical synovectomy in collagen-induced arthritis-affected rhesus monkeys. Hum Gene Ther 1999; 10:1139-1149.
83. Chen CC, Rivera A, Ron N et al. A gene therapy approach for treating T-cell-mediated autoimmune diseases. Blood 2001; 97:886-894.
84. Melo ME, Qian J, El-Amine M et al. Gene transfer of Ig-fusion proteins into B cells prevents and treats autoimmune diseases. J Immunol 2002; 168:4788-4795.
85. Jun HS, Chung YH, Han J et al. Prevention of autoimmune diabetes by immunogene therapy using recombinant vaccinia virus expressing glutamic acid decarboxylase. Diabetologia 2002; 45:668-676.
86. Melo ME, Qian J, El-Amine M et al. Gene transfer of Ig-fusion proteins into B cells prevents and treats autoimmune diseases. J Immunol 2002; 168:4788-4795.
87. Balasa B, Boehm BO, Fortnagel A et al. Vaccination with glutamic acid decarboxylase plasmid DNA protects mice from spontaneous autoimmune diabetes and B7/CD28 costimulation circumvents that protection. Clin Immunol 200; 99:241-252.
88. Galeano M, Deodato B, Altavilla D et al. Adeno-associated viral vector-mediated human vascular endothelial growth factor gene transfer stimulates angiogenesis and wound healing in the genetically diabetic mouse. Diabetologia 2003 [epub ahead of print].
89. Mahato RI, Henry J, Narang AS et al. Cationic lipid and polymer-based gene delivery to human pancreatic islets. Mol Ther 2003; 7:89-100.
90. Romano Di Peppe S, Mangoni A, Zambruno G et al. Adenovirus-mediated VEGF(165) gene transfer enhances wound healing by promoting angiogenesis in CD1 diabetic mice. Gene Ther 2002; 9:1271-1277.
91. Schratzberger P, Walter DH, Rittig K et al. Reversal of experimental diabetic neuropathy by VEGF gene transfer. J Clin Invest 2001; 107:1083-1092.
92. Rivard A, Silver M, Chen D et al. Rescue of diabetes-related impairment of angiogenesis by intramuscular gene therapy with adeno-VEGF. Am J Pathol 1999; 154:355-363.
93. Mathisen PM, Yu M, Yin L et al. Th2 T cells expressing transgene PDGF-α serve as vectors for gene therapy in autoimmune demyelinating disease. J Autoimm 1999; 3:31-38.
94. Yamasaki K, Edington HD, McClosky C et al. Reversal of impaired wound repair in iNOS-deficient mice by topical adenoviral-mediated iNOS gene transfer. J Clin Invest 1998; 101:967-971.
95. Ruffini F, Furlan R, Poliani PL et al. Fibroblast growth factor-II gene therapy reverts the clinical course and the pathological signs of chronic experimental autoimmune encephalomyelitis in C57BL/6 mice. Gene Ther 2001; 8:1207-1213.
96. Giannoukakis N, Mi Z, Rudert WA et al. Prevention of beta cell dysfunction and apoptosis activation in human islets by adenoviral gene transfer of the insulin-like growth factor I. Gene Ther 2000; 7:2015-2022.
97. Alam T, Sollinger HW. Glucose-regulated insulin production in hepatocytes. Transplantation 2002; 74:1781-1787.
98. Zhang W, Lu D, Kawazu S et al. Adenoviral Insulin Gene Therapy Prolongs Survival of IDDM Model BB Rats by Improving Hyperlipidemia. Horm Metab Res 2002; 34:577-582.
99. Martinenghi S, Cusella De Angelis G, Biressi S et al. Human insulin production and amelioration of diabetes in mice by electrotransfer-enhanced plasmid DNA gene transfer to the skeletal muscle. Gene Ther 2002; 9:1429-1437.
100. Jindal RM, Karanam M, Shah R. Prevention of diabetes in the NOD mouse by intra-muscular injection of recombinant adeno-associated virus containing the preproinsulin II gene. Int J Exp Diabetes Res 2001; 2:129-138.
101. Auricchio A, Gao GP, Yu QC et al. Constitutive and regulated expression of processed insulin following in vivo hepatic gene transfer. Gene Ther 2002; 9:963-971.
102. Shaw JA, Delday MI, Hart AW et al. Secretion of bioactive human insulin following plasmid-mediated gene transfer to non-neuroendocrine cell lines, primary cultures and rat skeletal muscle in vivo. J Endocrinol 2002; 172:653-672.
103. Dong H, Altomonte J, Morral N et al. Basal insulin gene expression significantly improves conventional insulin therapy in type 1 diabetic rats. Diabetes 2002; 51:130-138.

104. Nagamatsu S, Nakamichi Y, Ohara-Imaizumi M et al. Adenovirus-mediated preproinsulin gene transfer into adipose tissues ameliorates hyperglycemia in obese diabetic KKA(y) mice. FEBS Lett 2001; 509:106-110.
105. Shifrin AL, Auricchio A, Yu QC et al. Adenoviral vector-mediated insulin gene transfer in the mouse pancreas corrects streptozotocin-induced hyperglycemia. Gene Ther 2001; 8:1480-1489.
106. Yin D, Tang JG. Gene therapy for streptozotocin-induced diabetic mice by electroporational transfer of naked human insulin precursor DNA into skeletal muscle in vivo. FEBS Lett 2001; 495:16-20.
107. Chen R, Meseck ML, Woo SL. Auto-regulated hepatic insulin gene expression in type 1 diabetic rats. Mol Ther 2001; 3:584-590.
108. Chen R, Meseck M, McEvoy RC et al. Glucose-stimulated and self-limiting insulin production by glucose 6-phosphatase promoter driven insulin expression in hepatoma cells. Gene Ther 2000; 7:1802-1809.
109. Lee HC, Kim SJ, Kim KS et al. Remission in models of type 1 diabetes by gene therapy using a single-chain insulin analogue. Nature 2000; 408:483-488.
110. Thule PM, Liu JM. Regulated hepatic insulin gene therapy of STZ-diabetic rats. Gene Ther 2000; 7:1744-1752.
111. Morishita R, Gibbons GH, Kaneda Y et al. Systemic administration of HVJ viral coat-liposome complex containing human insulin vector decreases glucose level in diabetic mouse: A model of gene therapy. Biochem Biophys Res Commun 2000; 273:666-674.
112. Yamaguchi M, Kuzume M, Matsumoto T et al. Adenovirus-mediated insulin gene transfer improves nutritional and post-hepatectomized conditions in diabetic rats. Surgery 2000; 127:670-678.
113. Kon OL, Sivakumar S, Teoh KL et al. Naked plasmid-mediated gene transfer to skeletal muscle ameliorates diabetes mellitus. J Gene Med 1999; 1:186-194.
114. Falqui L, Martinenghi S, Severini GM et al. Reversal of diabetes in mice by implantation of human fibroblasts genetically engineered to release mature human insulin. Hum Gene Ther 1999;10:1753-1762.
115. Bochan MR, Shah R, Sidner RA et al. Reversal of diabetes in the rat by injection of hematopoietic stem cells infected with recombinant adeno-associated virus containing the preproinsulin II gene. Transplant Proc 1999; 31:690-691.
116. Shah R, Sidner RA, Bochan MR et al. Reversal of diabetes in streptozotocin-treated rats by intra muscular injection of recombinant adeno associated virus containing rat preproinsulin II gene. Transplant Proc 1999; 31:641-642.
117. Sugiyama A, Hattori S, Tanaka S et al. Defective adenoassociated viral-mediated transfection of insulin gene by direct injection into liver parenchyma decreases blood glucose of diabetic mice. Horm Metab Res 1997; 29:599-603.
118. Goldfine ID, German MS, Tseng HC et al. The endocrine secretion of human insulin and growth hormone by exocrine glands of the gastrointestinal tract. Nat Biotechnol 1997; 15:1378-1382.
119. Kasten-Jolly J, Aubrey MT, Conti DJ et al. Reversal of hyperglycemia in diabetic NOD mice by human proinsulin gene therapy. Transplant Proc 1997; 29:2216-2218.
120. Kolodka TM, Finegold M, Moss L et al. Gene therapy for diabetes mellitus in rats by hepatic expression of insulin. Proc Natl Acad Sci USA 1995; 92:3293-3297.
121. Taniguchi H, Nakauchi H, Iwata H et al. Treatment of diabetic mice with encapsulated fibroblasts producing human proinsulin. Transplant Proc 1992; 24:2977-2978.
122. Kawakami Y, Yamaoka T, Hirochika R et al. Somatic gene therapy for diabetes with an immunological safety system for complete removal of transplanted cells. Diabetes 1992; 41:956-961.
123. Flugel A, Matsumuro K, Neumann H et al. Anti-inflammatory activity of nerve growth factor in experimental autoimmune encephalomyelitis: inhibition of monocyte transendothelial migration. Eur J Immunol 2001; 31:11-22.
124. Goss JR, Goins WF, Lacomis D et al. Herpes simplex-mediated gene transfer of nerve growth factor protects against peripheral neuropathy in streptozotocin-induced diabetes in the mouse. Diabetes 2002; 51:2227-2232.
125. Goins WF, Yoshimura N, Phelan MW et al. Herpes simplex virus mediated nerve growth factor expression in bladder and afferent neurons: potential treatment for diabetic bladder dysfunction. J Urol 2001; 165:1748-1754.

126. Pradat PF, Kennel P, Naimi-Sadaoui S et al. Continuous delivery of neurotrophin 3 by gene therapy has a neuroprotective effect in experimental models of diabetic and acrylamide neuropathies. Hum Gene Ther 2001; 12:2237-2249.
127. Taniguchi H, Yamato E, Tashiro F et al. beta-cell neogenesis induced by adenovirus-mediated gene delivery of transcription factor pdx-1 into mouse pancreas. Gene Ther 2003; 10:15-23.
128. Kojima H, Fujimiya M, Matsumura K, NeuroD-betacellulin gene therapy induces islet neogenesis in the liver and reverses diabetes in mice. Nat Med 2003; 9:596-603.
129. Dobrzynski E, Montanari D, Agata J et al. Adrenomedullin improves cardiac function and prevents renal damage in streptozotocin-induced diabetic rats. Am J Physiol Endocrinol Metab 2002; 283:E1291-1298.
130. Morral N, McEvoy R, Dong H et al. Adenovirus-mediated expression of glucokinase in the liver as an adjuvant treatment for type 1 diabetes. Hum Gene Ther 2002; 13:1561-1570.
131. Emanueli C, Salis MB, Pinna A et al. Prevention of diabetes-induced microangiopathy by human tissue kallikrein gene transfer. Circulation 2002; 106:993-999.
132. Slosberg ED, Desai UJ, Fanelli B et al. Treatment of type 2 diabetes by adenoviral-mediated overexpression of the glucokinase regulatory protein. Diabetes 2001; 50:1813-1820.
133. Ozawa K, Kondo T, Hori O et al. Expression of the oxygen-regulated protein ORP150 accelerates wound healing by modulating intracellular VEGF transport. J Clin Invest 2001; 108:41-50.
134. Ueki K, Yamauchi T, Tamemoto H et al. Restored insulin-sensitivity in IRS-1-deficient mice treated by adenovirus-mediated gene therapy. J Clin Invest 2000; 105:1437-1445.
135. Yamasaki K, Edington HD, McClosky C et al. Reversal of impaired wound repair in iNOS-deficient mice by topical adenoviral-mediated iNOS gene transfer. J Clin Invest 1998; 101:967-971.
136. Murphy JE, Zhou S, Giese K et al. Long-term correction of obesity and diabetes in genetically obese mice by a single intramuscular injection of recombinant adeno-associated virus encoding mouse leptin. Proc Natl Acad Sci USA 1997; 94:13921-13926.
137. Muzzin P, Eisensmith RC, Copeland KC et al. Correction of obesity and diabetes in genetically obese mice by leptin gene therapy. Proc Natl Acad Sci USA 1996; 93:14804-14808.
138. van der Laan WH, Quax PH, Seemayer CA et al. Cartilage degradation and invasion by rheumatoid synovial fibroblasts is inhibited by gene transfer of TIMP-1 and TIMP-3. Gene Ther 2003; 10:234-242.
139. Martino G, Furlan R, Comi G et al. The ependymal route to the CNS: an emerging gene-therapy approach for MS. Trends Immunol 2001; 22:483-490.
140. http://www.wiley.co.uk/wileychi/genmed/clinical/, trial no. 357.
141. http://www.wiley.co.uk/wileychi/genmed/clinical/, trial no. 627.

CHAPTER 2

Gene Therapeutics in Autoimmune Diabetes

Jon D. Piganelli, Massimo Trucco and Nick Giannoukakis*

Overview of Therapeutic Challenges in Type 1 Diabetes Mellitus (T1D)

A significant amount of resources has recently been devoted to the restoration of normal glycemic regulation in type 1 diabetic patients by transplantation of allogeneic islets of Langerhans. Despite the promise offered by this approach, logistical hurdles necessitate a comprehensive strategy aimed at different molecular and cellular determinants of the autoimmune pathology of type 1 diabetes. Developments in gene therapy permit the engineering of immune cells, islets, surrogate beta cells as well as the conditioning of the transplant recipient in order to facilitate allograft survival. More importantly, manipulation of subsets of immune cells also offers an opportunity to intervene prophylactically and within the short time-span between clinical diagnosis and complete beta cell mass destruction to restore some degree of normoglycemia. While outlining the issues that challenge the translatability of gene therapeutics to the diabetic clinic, we give an overview of the exciting potential that such gene therapeutic strategies can offer the clinician.

Molecular and Cellular Determinants of Type 1 Diabetes in Mouse and Man

T1D is considered a classical autoimmune disease that is characterized by a breakdown in both central and peripheral tolerance. The breakdown in central tolerance leads to precursor pools of self-reactive T cells that escape into the periphery. In the periphery, an immune response against the pancreatic beta cells is inititiated by as yet-unknown environmental triggers, ultimately leading to beta cell destruction and diabetes.[1,2] In the nonobese diabetic (NOD) mouse,[3] the most widely used animal model of T1D; the defect in peripheral tolerance is evident because the NOD suffers from spontaneous autoimmune diabetes.[4,5] However, a very important study by Markees et al[6] suggests that NOD mice have an inherent defect in peripheral tolerance, demonstrated by the inability of anti-CD40-treatment to induced tolerance to skin allografts, a tissue to which NOD mice have no known autoimmune reactivity. Furthermore, it has been demonstrated that NOD mice display enhanced immune responses and prolonged survival of lymphoid cells when immunized with nominal antigens.[7] These data support the paradigm that the NOD mouse may have peripheral tolerance defects that go

*Nick Giannoukakis—Department of Pathology, University of Pittsburgh School of Medicine, Diabetes Institute, Rangos Research Center, 3460 Fifth Avenue, Pittsburgh, Pennsylvania 15213, U.S.A. Email: ngiann1@pitt.edu

Gene Therapy of Autoimmune Disease, edited by Gérald J. Prud'homme. ©2005 Eurekah.com and Kluwer Academic / Plenum Publishers.

beyond the manifestation of autoimmunity that also render these mice resistant to conventional allograft tolerizing strategies as well as exacerbated immune activation upon any antigenic challenge. Thus it appears that the "rules" governing peripheral tolerance in autoimmune prone individuals are vastly different or more rigorous than those that impact nonautoimmune individuals. Therefore if autoimmune-prone individuals have inherently stringent requirements for tolerance induction, then such recipients may require strategic design in therapies including, combinatorial therapies, in order to achieve successful treatment both prophylactically as well as for allograft transplant tolerance.

Studies conducted in the NOD mouse have determined that the infiltrate within the islets is composed of $CD4^+$, $CD8^+$, T lymphocytes, B-lymphocytes, macrophages, and dendritic cells.[8-11] The T cell subsets play an obligatory role in the initiation of the disease. In the NOD mouse it has been demonstrated that CD8 T cells are critical for the initiation of disease progression, while the CD4 population is indispensable for the mobilization of the mononuclear cell infiltrate. Although $CD8^+$ T cells are critical in the diabetes process, $CD8^+$ T cells isolated from stock NOD mice cannot independently initiate Type I diabetes.[8,12,13] Thus it appears that the $CD8^+$ T cell population that contributes to T1D development, in the stock NOD mouse, is dependent on helper functions provided by $CD4^+$ T cells.[14] This may be due to a $CD4^+$ dependent expansion of $CD8^+$ T cells to critical threshold levels, which can then initiate pathogenic effects. The $CD4^+$ and $CD8^+$ TCR transgenic mouse models that express a TCR from diabetogenic clones support this concept of critical expansion for initiation of disease. Both $CD4^+$ [15] and $CD8^+$ [14] TCR-transgenic strains can, independently of the either T cell subtype initiate diabetes. Clearly, the coordinate interaction of both the innate and adaptive immune response is necessary for the development of disease.

A large body of evidence supports the concept that the antigen specific, T cell-mediated infiltration of inflammatory cells to the pancreas leads to the generation of reactive oxygen species (ROS), {superoxide, (O_2^-), hydroxyl radical (^-OH), nitric oxide (NO^-) and peroxynitrite ($ONOO^-$)}, and pro-inflammatory cytokines (TNFα, IL-1β and IFNγ).[16-18] Synergistic interaction between ROS and these cytokines results in the ultimate destruction of the pancreatic beta cells by both apoptotic and necrotic cell death. There is an extensive literature on the effect of free oxygen and nitric oxide radicals elaborated either by infiltrating immune cells or as a result of cytokine-induced beta cell-specific expression of enzymes generating these radicals (inducible nitric oxide synthase). Locally produced ROS are involved in the effector mechanisms of beta cell destruction.[16-21] In vitro, T cell and macrophage cytokines such as IFNγ, IL-1β and TNFα induce the production of ROS by beta cells, which leads to beta cell destruction.[22] This destruction may ultimately be caused by an apoptotic mechanism.[23-27] Beta cells engineered to over-express antioxidant proteins have been shown to be resistant to ROS and NO[5,28-30] Furthermore, stable expression of manganese superoxide dismutase (Mn-SOD) in insulinoma cells prevented IL-1β-induced cytotoxicity and reduced nitric oxide production.[29] Finally, others have shown that transgenic mice with beta cell-targeted over-expression of copper, zinc SOD or thioredoxin have increased resistance to autoimmune and streptozotocin-induced diabetes.[31-33] The protective effects demonstrated with the use of stable expression of antioxidant genes was recapitulated through the use of a superoxide dismutase mimic (a small molecule antioxidant) in an adoptive transfer system of autoimmune diabetes by a diabetogenic $CD4^+$ T cell clone.[34,35] These results are particularly exciting, as they are consistent with the previous reports where vector-mediated or transgenic over-expression of anti-oxidants protected beta cells. The ability to protect beta cells against CD4 mediated generation of pro-inflammatory cytokines and free radicals through the use of antioxidant therapy support the model of free radical generation as a pathogenic mechanism of T1D.

While less precise and specific data exist for the actual mechanism of beta cell destruction in humans, the body of evidence points to similarities between the etiopathology in the NOD mouse and humans. The chronic onset, the presence of a cellular inflammation, the transferability of diabetes and of protection by bone marrow transplantation and the immunosuppressibility by conventional pharmacologic agents. The genetics of the disease is multifactorial in humans and in the NOD mouse.[36-38] In humans, two loci (IDDM1 and IDDM2) have been confirmed to be in linkage with the disease. IDDM1 encompasses the HLA gene complex and it alone defines the most important risk factor. In humans the disease is associated with the inheritance of DR3/DR4 haplotypes (DR3: DQA1*0501, DQB1*0201 and DR4: DQA1*0301, DQB1*0302.[39,40] IDDM2 has been mapped to a variable number of tandem repeats (VNTR) polymorphism upstream of the insulin gene promoter which can determine thymic levels of insulin.[41,42] In fact, a recent study demonstrated that the number of active copies of insulin in a transgenic mouse can influence the degree of immune cell reactivity towards insulin, a putative autoantigen.[43] A number of other loci have demonstrated suggestive associations, but to date, none of these results have been replicated to establish significant linkage with the disease.[44-46]

A number of earlier hypotheses with some supporting evidence have been put forward to explain the possible mechanism of action of the environmental trigger including beta cell death secondary to virally-triggered inflammation, molecular mimicry, superantigens and diet.[47-50] [51-56] What is certain is that at some point post-natally, the immune system of a genetically-predisposed individual is activated to chronically infiltrate the islets of Langerhans. While the initial phase of infiltration may not involve beta cell destruction, a number of studies in vivo and in vitro suggest that immune cells become able to render beta cells dysfunctional through the actions of cytokines they produce.

Therapeutic Options

Other than insulin replacement by daily injections of the hormone, the only other clinically-acceptable means of insulin restoration remains islet transplantation.[57-60] Recent advances in understanding transplantation immunology in general and the process of insulitis and the molecular/genetic bases of failure of central and/or peripheral mechanisms of tolerance to tissue-restricted antigens in particular have yielded a number of approaches for therapy and prevention ofT1D. To manipulate the immune system in a prophylactic manner, cell and gene based modalities or a combination of both were tested. Therapeutic strategies strive instead to improve islet transplantation by improving insulin secretion, engraftment and most importantly, protection of the transplant from allogeneic immune rejection. In humans, islet grafts derive from allogeneic cadaveric donors. Stem/progenitor cells, alone or in engineered form are also potential candidates for beta cell replacement. Each approach has shown promise, but each approach has also demonstrated its limitations. New data suggest that a critical period between time of diagnosis and actual destruction of beta cell mass required for appropriate glycemic control (the so-called "honeymoon period"; see below) may be exploited immunologically to obviate the need of islet transplantation altogether. While antibody-based approaches are currently being tested, it is anticipated that emerging gene and cell therapies can overcome the safety and negative systemic effects associated with the antibody approach.

Insulin Replacement: Islets or Surrogate Beta Cells

Novel immunosuppressive cocktails, culture in the presence of homologous serum proteins, minimization of time between pancreas procurement and islet processing combined with transplantation of a larger beta cell mass, were the most significant steps in improving islet transplantation outcome in the studies of Shapiro et al.[61-64] Although it is not clear which of the parameters contributed the most to success, many factors still limit a large-scale diffusion of islet and beta cell replacement for type 1 diabetic patients. The need for chronic immunosuppression and for multiple donors as a source for islets remain the prime reasons or factors which impose a search for alternative ways of promoting islet cell allograft survival. Tolerogenic protocols, once successful, may allow the use of islet transplantation in young diabetic patients.

Gene transfer technology is such an option and a number of advances have been attained in animal models of islet allograft transplantation. Table 1 lists experiments in which significant prolongation of islet allograft or xenograft survival has been achieved.

The main obstacle for a gene transfer-based approach is the choice of gene transfer vectors. Despite initial enthusiasm about the versatility of adenoviral vectors, their inherent immunogenicity raises a number of serious concerns in view of their possible application to engineer human islets for clinical use. The advent of lentiviral vectors appeared to alleviate some of the immunogenicity concerns, but lentivirus are not as efficient as adenoviruses in transducing intact human islets. Tables 2 to 4 list a number of gene transfer vectors as well as their pros and cons in the context of gene transfer to intact islets. However, an under-appreciated factor that very likely affects the success of islet engraftment is the metabolic status of the islets themselves following isolation and culture. There is no doubt that the time between organ retrieval and islet processing with the ineherent intermediate steps including cold storage and enzymatic/mechanical digestion, affects islet yield, viability and function.[35,65] Furthermore the culture conditions prior to transplantation can crucially affect islet cells physiology and, consequently, the chance of successful engraftment. In general, the cessation of the oxygen supply to the pancreatic tissue at the time of donor organ harvesting, is known to trigger ischemic damage, free-radical mediated cell degeneration as well as initiation of apoptosis.[66,67] Also, the separation of the islets from the surrounding matrix and from the neighbor cells driven by the isolation procedure, further contributes to activate cell apoptosis.[68,69] Immediate-onset ischemia has been proposed to be an important determinant of acute and chronic allograft rejection.[70] In addition, organs carrying contaminating immune and a large number of endothelial cells or in which platelets have been trapped, will likely experience a so-called "cytokine storms", where the onset of apoptototic processes causes an abnormally large release of stored cytokines and other proinflammatory soluble mediators. Moreover a cycle is initiated whereby cytokines release can exacerbate the formation of reactive oxygen intermediates.[71] Presumably the combination of all these mechanisms predispose the islets to environmental damage both during culture and at the transplantation site, where inflammation is likely to occur shortly after implant even before allo-immune response initiates. Potential approaches to avoid this situation can include the perfusion of the organs with solutions containing chemical inhibitors of apoptosis (ZVAD-fmk) as well as anti-apoptotic genes like bcl-2,bcl-xL, and enzymes that break down, or prevent, the formation of free-radicals such as catalase, thioredoxin, heme-oxigenase-1 and superoxide dismutase.[72-77] Some of these anti-apoptotic proteins fused to protein-transduction domains can successfully prevent apoptosis and significantly improve islet yield and survival following isolation.[34,65,78] We and others have also shown that the inclusion of synthetic mimetics of free-redical scavengers seem to prevent islet degeneration possibly limiting the initiation of apoptotic processes.[34,35] Islets also take up oligonucleotides quite efficiently (unpublished observations). Knowledge of the primary transcripts whose protein products are involved in apoptosis activation or suppression of insulin production can be targeted with antisense oligonucleotides during the isolation procedure.

Oligonucleotide therapy offers a simple and convenient method to interfere with not only gene expression, but also with transcription using short double-stranded decoys containing binding sites for specific transcription factors involved in inflammatory responses, like NF-kB and STATs. Soluble binding proteins and ligand-binding domains of chemokines can also be considered potential tools with which primary islet dysfunction can be prevented. Chemokines are potent immunoattractants fairly resistant to degradation and are sequestered by proteoglycans

Table 1. Target genes for the therapy of diabetes

A. Genes which promote islet allo-/xenograft survival in vitro and in vivo and/or beta cell survival in culture

Anti-apoptotic genes
- bcl-2[74,75,234-236]
- bcl-xL[78,237]
- heme oxygenase-1[72,73,238]
- dominant negative protein kinase C delta[239]
- dominant negative MyD88[240]
- IGF-I[241]
- IkappaB alpha super-repressor[242]
- Hsp70[243]
- A20[244]
- PEA-15[78]
- catalase[245,246]
- manganese superoxide dismutase[247]
- I-kappaB kinase inhibitor[248]

Cytokines:
- IL-4[249] (although one report demonstrated no protection[250])
- interleukin-1 receptor antagonist protein[251]
- IL-12p40[252]
- viral IL-10[253]
- IL-10[254] (one report did not show protection[250])
- TGF-beta[254] (one report showed negative results[255])

Immunoregulatory genes:
- Indoleamine 2,3-dioxygenase[256]
- CTLA-4Ig[257]
- Fas ligand[258] (although in a number of reports Fas ligand was not protective:[259])
- adenoviral E3 genes[260]

B. Other gene/cell therapy approaches to prevent/abrogate autoimmunity and/or promote islet allo-/xenograft survival

Bone marrow transplantation/chimerism induction[183,188-191,222,261-266]

Antigen-presenting cell transfer
- class I MHC[267]
- autologous dendritic cell transfer[193]

Co-stmulation blockade
- soluble ICAM-1-Ig[268]
- CTLA-4Ig[269-273]
- OX40Ig[272]

Cytokines
- IL-10[274-277]
- IL-4[275,278]
- soluble IFN-gamma receptor[279,280]
- TGF-beta[281]
- VIL-10[277]

Autoantigen transfer
- GAD[282,283]

Others
- adenovirus E3 proteins[284]
- orally-administered putative autoantigens (insulin, GAD)[285-287]
- CD152[288]

Table 2. Gene vectors which transduce islets (with references)

Plasmid DNA [257,289-291]
Adenovirus [244,250,252,253,258,260,292-299]
Adeno-associated virus [74,75,89,91,241,242,251,256,300-304]
MoLV retrovirus [305]
Lentivirus [249,306,307]
Herpes simplex virus [234,235]
Cationic liposomes [290,291,295]
Peptide fusion domains [78,248,308]

Table 3. Properties of gene transfer vectors with applicability to islet gene transfer

Vector Type	Stable Transduction	Cell Cycle Requirements	Immunogenicity	Islets Transduced?
Plasmid DNA	No	Dividing/non-dividing	No	Mouse/human
Adenovirus	No	Dividing/non-dividing	Yes	Mouse/human
Adeno-associated virus	Possibly	Dividing/non-dividing	Minor	Human
MoLV-based retrovirus	Yes	Dividing	No	(Mouse/human) Very poor
Lentivirus	Yes	Dividing/non-dividing	No	Mouse/human
Herpes simplex type-1 virus	No	Dividing/non-dividing	Inherent toxicity	Human
Cationic liposome	No	Dividing/non-dividing	No	Human
Peptide fusion domains	No	Dividing/non-dividing	No	Human/mouse

on the endothelium.[79,80] Chemokines promote endothelial adhesion in addition to their chemotaxin properties.[79,80] Virally-encoded proteins have been identified which bind chemokines and could be a means of achieveing chemokine blockade.[81,82] This blockade can easily be attained using peptide transduction domains fused to recombinant proteins or short oligonucleotides, especially if administered during procurement and reperfusion of the donor pancreas. However, long-term expression of some of these molecules may have a greater effect on graft survival once stable gene expression is achieved. This necessitates the use of gene vectors that can deliver the therapeutic gene with the objective of expression for the entire lifetime of the recipient.

Injection of animals with a number of vectors like adenovirus[83-88] and adeno-associated virus[89-92] encoding proinsulin under the control of a number of promoters including CMV, insulin, PEPCK and L-pyruvate kinase has resulted in correction of hyperglycemia. In many instances, however, the effect appears to have been transient. This approach suffers from the potential immunogenicity of the virus and in many cases precludes a second dosing due to the generation of neutralizing antibodies. Other issues are related to choice of promoter, which in the instance of L-pyruvate kinase demonstrates slow kinetics, although one study with this promoter was able to achieve relatively rapid responses to glucose.[90] Finally, many tissues do not express the necessary proteinases which process proinsulin into the potent bioactive insulin.

Table 4. General characteristics of gene delivery vehicles

Vector Type	Pros	Cons
Plasmid DNA	Easy to engineer, grow and purify; multicistronic variants easy to engineer	Poor persistence, non-specific cell targeting, poor tissue diffusion
Adenovirus	Choice vector for pilot proof-of-principle experiments; High titers easily obtained; almost all cells and tissues are transducible; cell retargeting is possible	Immunogenic in vivo; non-stable transduction
Adeno-associated virus	Site-specific, stable integration achievable, almost absent immunogenicity; many cell types transducible	Time for transgene expression can be on the order of days
MoLV-based retrovirus	Stably integrating vector in rapidly-dividing cells; cell-type retargeting possible; good titers obtainable	Subject to chromosomal position—effect sensitivity of—as well as methylation and cytokine effects on gene expression
Lentivirus	Non-immunogenic, stablyintegrating; Choice vector for non-dividing, non-cycling cells; good titers obtainable; Data support absence of replication-competent-recombinant vector particles in stocks	Clinical safety concerns with HIV-1-based vectors
Herpes simplex type-1 virus	Large genome available for multiple large size cistrons; good persistence in many cell types; cell-type retargeting possible	Inherent toxicity
Cationic liposome	Easy to manipulate to deliver plasmid DNA to almost all cells and tissue. Non-immunogenic; cell-type non-specific, cell-type retargeting possible	Poor control of diffusion kinetics
Peptide fusion domains	Many cell-types transducible; High-level protein/peptide import; intact proteins/ peptides delivered; not subject to gene regulation; targeting of specific proteins possible; high-level peptide production easily achievable; no reported immunogenicity	Short half life; subject to proteolytic degradation; large amounts require some time to generate

Beta Cell Surrogates

Surrogate beta cells offer an alternative to intact islet transplantation and direct injection of proinsulin-expressing vectors. A variety of cell types including fibroblasts, muscle, neuroendocrine cells and hepatocytes have been engineered to produce insulin.[93-97] Despite these exciting data, a very recent manuscript considers alternative hypotheses for the observations made and cautions in favor of very stringent experimentation to make the conclusion that nonbeta cells can produce and express insulin.[98] In contrast, the most notable advances have been made using engineered hepatocytes.[85,87,88] Hepatocytes are particularly attractive because they can easily engraft in the liver, and because they possess identical glucose-sensing molecules as the pancreas (e.g., GLUT2, GK). Furthermore, one can exploit a number of hepatocyte gene promoters which are sensitive to glucose, in order to engineer insulin transgenes to be glucose concentration-sensitive. Despite a number of promising approaches exploiting a number of glucose-regulated promoters,[85,90,99-106] much more work is needed to make hepatocytes into fully surrogate beta cells. The first feature that a hepatocyte is missing to properly act like a beta cell surrogate is the ability to respond to glucose in a sufficiently rapid fashion, as rapid as that characteristic of beta cells. Second, the liver-specific glucose-sensitive promoters have elements that respond to hormonal and metabolic signals which can impede, attenuate or abrogate the desired objective of tight glucose regulation. For example, instances of hyperglucagonemia which is to be expected in the absence of functional endogenous beta cells in diabetics, will most likely attenuate or repress the LPK promoter as well as other promoters such as glucokinase.[88,107,108] Third, glucose-dependent trans-activation of the LPK promoter requires GK-dependent phosphorylation of glucose, an activity that is insulin-dependent[103]). Other promoters have been suggested, such as that of phosphoenolcarboxykinase (PEPCK), but this promoter is activated by glucagon and inhibited by insulin, which may not result in the desired kinetics of physiological gluco-regulation.[109,110] It is possible that a combination of promoter elements from different glucose-responive hepatic genes may be needed to create an optimal synthetic promoter to drive hepatic insulin expression in a true glucose-sensitive fashion.

In an entirely different approach, tissue-specific promoters have been exploited to engineer cells to express insulin in cells that are not targets of autoimmune destruction. Lipes et al have expressed insulin in the anterior pituitary gland of NOD mice under the control of the pro-opiomelanocortin promoter. Insulin was expressed, stored into secretory granules and exhibited regulated secretion. Moreover, transplantation of transgenic anterior pituitary tissue to NOD mice was able to partially restore normoglycemia without any signs of immune rejection.[111,112] It was not clear however, if in these cells, insulin secretion was glucose concentration-dependent. More recently, an ingenious approach harnessing intestinal K-cells as surrogate glucose-responsive insulin producers was demonstrated. In this approach, transgenic mice expressing human insulin under the control of the gastrointestinal inhibitory peptide (GIP) promoter were generated. These mice expressed and secreted insulin from intestinal K cells in which the GIP promoter is active. Insulin secretion in these mice was glucose-responsive and was maintained following streptozotocin treatment, indicating that the K-cells were spared the effects of streptozotocin.[113] These data suggest that it may be feasible to target the intestinal cells with vectors encoding the GIP-Insulin transgene, or by ex vivo engineering intestinal cells in which glucose-sensitive promoters are driving insulin expression. However, an effective means of gene delivery to these cells needs to be developed for in vivo gene therapy, as these cells are present in the crypts of the gut, significantly impeding access to viral transduction.

Stem and Progenitor Cells

The considerable genetic manipulations that are required to convert nonbeta cells into efficient glucose-sensing, insulin-secreting cells have led other investigators into considering means of expanding adult or neonatal beta cells or of harnessing the developmental potential of islet precursor cells and of embryonal stem cells. However, despite the culture conditions and manipulations, commitment to beta cells and insulin production has not always been consistent.[114-119] Much excitement has also surrounded observations that adult stem cells from bone marrow or from other tissues could "transdifferentiate" into a number of other lineage-different cell types. Such stem cells have been described and sometimes physically isolated in the nervous system, pancreas, epidermis, mesenchyme, liver, bone, muscle and endothelium. Hematopoietic stem cells, in some studies were proven able to yield endothelial, brain, muscle, liver and mesenchymal cells. In some studies, hematopoietic cells could also be generated from neuronal or muscle stem cells (reviewed in ref. 120). A number of issues however, have tempered the enthusiasm with which these observations were initially greeted. The contamination of hematopoietic stem cells with mesenchymal precursors, or the programming by growth factors in culture, and more recently, the phenomenon of fusion of stem cells with tissue cells and false positives due to insulin in the culture media are perhaps the most important variables to better test.[98,120,121] Recent developments, however, strengthen the belief that mesenchymal cells in bone marrow may be a multipotent source of cells.[122-124] This characteristic can be exploited, however there are no data on whether such cells can be differentiated along the islet and beta cell lineage. Clearly, the ability to manipulate blood-borne progenitors into the beta cell lineage should provide a significant breakthrough for surrogate beta cell technology as insulin replacement.

Despite the current controversy and the serious ethical issues raised by cloning technology, it is likely that therapeutic cloning, under strict and defined conditions, will find its place in stem cell therapies.[125-127] In this regard, one possible means of propagating beta cells or progenitors while avoiding the complications involved with the immune response could entail the removal of DNA or nucleus from somatic cells of a patient, transfer it into an enucleated embryonal stem cell and its expansion into an appropriate beta cell lineage. While this remains highly speculative at present, the rapid pace of basic work in this area, despite restrictions, will likely yiel insight into such manipulations.

Immortalization of islet cells with a beta cell phenotype has been attempted and successfully achieved. Insulin production, however, seems to be linked to terminal differentiation of the cell, an event normally reached with growth arrest. This problem has so far limited the utility of cell immortalization. Also, this approach carries with it the possibility of oncogenic transformation.[128-131]

Although still controversial, there are data indicating that mature human beta cells can be induced to replicate under the effects of hepatocyte growth factor (HGF).[132-134] The limitation of this approach, however, rests on the loss of differentiation of the induced beta cell along with a substantial decrease in insulin production.[135] Conditional replication of nonhuman beta cells has been achieved by placing the SV-40 T antigen under the control of an inducible promoter.[129] In these studies, beta cells were able to replicate and to maintain differentiated function under inducible conditions. No data exist on whether such an approach is feasible in human beta cells.

Propagation of islet precursor cells with subsequent genetic manipulation to commit them to the beta cell lineage and ultimately to beta cells has also been considered.[118,136] To become feasible, this approach, however, requires a more complete understanding of the hierarchy of master regulatory transcriptional genes. Depending upon the cell type, PDX-1 over-expression can impart onto it a beta cell or a beta-cell-like phenotype.[137-139] Indeed, Ferber et al demonstrated that adenoviral gene transfer of a PDX-1 gene into liver resulted in insulin-expressing cells, although it was not clear if these cells were glucose-sensitive and were actually secreting the insulin in a timely fashion.[140] Other important transcriptional regulators associated with differentiation of ductal epithelial cells into endocrine islet cells include the HNF family of transcription factors, PAX-4 and PAX-6, NeuroD/B2, Nkx 2.2 and Nkx 6.1.[141-143] Along with intracellular determinants, precursor cells require signalling from their environment to differentiate appropriately. A variety of polypeptide growth factors including insulin-like growth factors I and II,[144-148] prolactin,[149] placental lactogen,[150,151] parathyroid hormone-related peptide,[152,153] and to a limited extent, TGF-alpha,[154-156] can promote pancreatic cell growth and islet cell proliferation. Hart and colleagues have produced evidence suggesting that fibroblast growth factor (FGF) signalling is important for beta cell generation.[157,158] Strategies aimed at engineering beta cell progenitors from pancreatic ductular epithelium with FGF in the presence of a permissive PDX-1 expression could promote expansion of beta cell progentors or a differentiation of progenitors into a prebeta cell lineage.

Another class of factors has been identified whose expression and production is associated with pancreatic regeneration.[159-161] The Reg secreted protein, in particular, promotes increases in beta cell mass in rats that had undergone pancreatectomy.[162-164] The expression and secretion of another molecule that belongs to the Reg family of proteins, termed INGAP (islet neogenesis associated protein), is upregulated in hamster islets where neogenesis was artificially induced.[165,166] The precise role of INGAP on beta cell proliferation and function, however, remains unclear.

Bonner-Weir and colleagues have shown that it may be feasible to derive beta cell cluster buds from exocrine pancreatic tissue from which originate the ductular epithelial cells destined to become endocrine pancreatic islet cells.[167] This approach is exciting in that mature, nonendocrine tissue of the pancreas need not be wasted during the process of islet isolation, but can be used in defined culture systems to generate islet progenitor cells for further manipulation, genetic or hormonal.

Thus, taken together, the transfer of combinations of genes encoding soluble and intracellular differentiation factors to stem/progenitor cells could become feasible once their precise role in the pathway of commitment and differentiation to beta cells becomes clearer. However, beta cells have a limited life-span in vitro. To what extent apoptosis or senescence play a role in this is uncertain. Nonetheless, a better understanding of cell cycle control in beta cells or neonatal islet cells could lead to the discovery of molecules that could be exploited, in a conditional manner, to promote growth in vivo and maintenance or extension of life-span, both in vitro and in vivo. Possible means include the transfer of cyclin-dependent kinases, pro-replication and mitotic factors and/or telomerase, to promote expanded cell life-span, all under regulatable promoters. Such an approach could achieve the expansion of semi-committed or fully committed islet precursor cells, or early beta cells. Combined with xenogeneic donor manipulation, these interventions could provide an almost limitless supply of beta cells for transplantation. The recent success in knocking in a nonfunctional α1,3)-galactosyltransferase in order to generate a transgenic pig deficient for this enzyme, may forecast the inclusion of modalities in which transgenic porcine islets can be used instead of allogeneic human islets for transplantation.[168-170] The importance of this breakthrough is underscored by the fact that the major target of xenoreactive antibodies which promote an acute rejection of porcine tissues is the epitope that is synthesized by this enzyme. While this is the major porcine xenoantigen, it is almost certain that other minor porcine epitopes will contribute, perhaps not to acute rejection, but to delayed or chronic xenograft rejection and these are challenges that must be surmounted in the future.

The Gene Vehicles: Viral, Nonviral and Cellular

An appreciable amount of work has focused on using viral vectors to infect intact islets in culture prior to transplantation into recipients to impede the allogeneic rejection (reviewed in Giannoukakis et al[171,172]). The excitement generated by these studies, however, was tempered by the appreciation that permanent allograft survival was generally not achieved. Often, to explain this limited success, investigators invoke the immunogenicity of the particular vector used, although recent evidence suggests that the quality of the islets may be more crucial than the vector choice in determining the presence and grade of inflammation in and around the graft.[65] Tables 2 to 4 list the vectors that have been used to date to transduce intact human islets as well as their pros and cons. The list indirectly demonstrates that no "ideal" vector yet exists. New technology including small interference RNA (siRNA),[173] adeno-associated virus inverted terminal repeat (AAV ITR)-based plasmids,[174,175] novel classes of lentivirus (EIAV, FIV),[176-182] lentivirus-herpesvirus hybrids and other viral vectors, is in development, but their efficiency has yet to be reported in the context of intact islet transduction. Equally unknown is the degree to which these vectors can contribute to post-transplantation inflammation.

Cell therapy constitutes an alternative approach to induce tolerance to alloantigens. Allogeneic bone marrow transplantation, with or without the addition of immunoregulatory antibodies (blocking CD28:B7 and CD40:CD40 ligand interactions), has been the choice of many investigators to promote allogeneic islet transplantation in mouse models of autoimmune diabetes.[183-192] In some instances, permanent allograft survival has been reported in prediabetic mice (permanent in the sense that the recipient maintained normoglycemia at the time it was last tested). It is not clear however, if these strategies would work equally well in an already-diabetic individual. A number of studies attempted to promote the activity of regulatory immune cells by dendritic cells. This novel and rational approach, however, may require multiple administrations to maintain a sufficient level of activity.[193,194] Combinations of these approaches, including gene-engineered dendritic cells expressing a variety of immunosuppressive molecules have shown promise in allograft survival[195-201] and are awaiting rigorous testing in the context of islet allograft transplantation. Considering successes and failures, it is perhaps fair to conclude that while gene vectors and cells alone may not have yet supported permanent islet allograft survival, their utility cannot be yet dismissed as many important parameters have still to be evaluated, including combinative approaches. In fact, very few studies have attempted to engineer islets expressing more than one immunoregulatory transgene at a time. This is an important aspect of the problem to consider since the immune response against the transplant (and perhaps the vector) may involve more than one pathway.

Prevention Strategies

In order to prevent the disorder, one must be able to first identify with a sufficient degree of confidence individuals who are at very high risk for developing type 1 diabetes. While inheritance of susceptibility alleles at loci linked to and/or associated with the disorder is an important risk factor, it alone cannot guarantee that the individual will in fact become diabetic. This is the main reason for the ongoing debates on prevention based on genetic screening.[39,202] While outright prevention based only on genetic screening may not be yet acceptable, other strategies which fall inside the realm of "prevention" can be acceptable. There are data indicating that newly-onset diabetics still possess adequate beta cell mass to sustain normoglycemia if the autoimmune inflammation can be promptly controlled.[203-209] The time between diagnosis and elimination of beta cell mass adequate to sustain normoglycemia has been termed the "honeymoon" period. One can exploit immunoregulatory networks to promote hyporesponsiveness of autoaggressive immune cells in this period as a viable means of improving or restoring normoglycemia. Supporting this approach are the studies where treatment of prediabetic and/or overtly-diabetic NOD mice with an anti-CD3 antibody restored normoglycemia in a substantial portion of mice for a sustained period of time.[210] Very recently, human trials using the same approach also seem quite promising.[211] Although clinical diabetes onset has most often been associated with beta cell death, it is possible that the the low levels of insulin production are due to the effects of cytokines which modulate their production. If this is the case, this process can be reversed.[212-218] Some data strongly suggest that suppression of the activity of the insulitic cells by the induction of immune hyporesponsiveness in clinically-diabetic individuals may promote either beta cell neogenesis and/or rescue of the cytokine-suppressed beta cells in the insulitic environment.[192]

Inherent in this philosophy is the ability to promote T1D-specific autoantigen tolerance or T1D-specific autoantigen immune hyporesponsiveness. To acheieve this, one can target genes and/or cells to the thymus, or one can manipulate the peripheral immune effectors using cells alone or gene-engineered cells. The evidence suggesting that a preventive approach manipulating the thymic environment of antigen presentation is possible was initially obtained by generating transgenic NOD mice with different H2 genes. Mice carrying H2 transgenes conferring resistance did not develop diabetes.[219,220] Additionally, diabetes in the NOD mouse was also prevented by thymic inoculation of soluble islet antigens in the form of cellular lysates or by expression of putative beta cell autoantigens in the thymus.[219,221] Could this approach be clinically-applicable? Recent data on plasticity of bone marrow stem cells[120,122-124] seem to imply that culture conditions could be defined in which bone marrow progenitors could be propagated towards "thymic" antigen-presenting cells. These cells could be engineered using a number of viral or nonviral vector methods (gene vectors to be described in a later section) to present autoantigen. These cells could then be injected into the host where they could eventually populate the recipient thymus. To obviate the problems associated with graft versus host disease in an allogeneic context, one could envisage the use of hematopoietic stem cells propagated from peripheral blood precursors of the recipient. Preliminary evidence seems to suggest that the newly-generated insulin-generating cells may not have the same phenotypic makeup of normal beta cells and because of this characteristic, they may be able to escape the recurrence of preexisting autoimmunity.

A number of studies have shown that allogeneic bone marrow transplantation into NOD or BB rats with the aim of inducing a state of chimerism can also prevent diabetes and facilitate allo- and xenograft islet transplantation.[183-192,222] While the mechanisms are believed to involve central and peripheral tolerance, the applicability of this approach in humans is impeded by the use of very high radiation conditioning of the recipient. The need for complete or partial myeloablative treatment and of allogeneic donors could be obviated by genetically-engineering peripheral blood-derived autologous hematopoietic stem cells with transgenes promoting the induction and activity of immunoregulatory networks. Independently of the means utilized to abrogate autoimmunity, a state in which the diabetic patient is free of autoreactive T-cells and their assault on pancreatic beta cells is optimal to allow or promote the rescue or regeneration of enough insulin-secreting cells in the endogenous pancreas. This may allow physiologic euglycemia. Alternative measures to control the glycemia during the possibly long recovery period must also be implemented.

Although considered potent immunostimulators, dendritic cells (DC) have recently been shown to possess tolerogenic characteristics under defined conditions. DC tolerogenicity manifested as the suppression of T cell activation, has been documented in tumor, allo-, and auto-immunity.[223] The conditions that can yield tolerogenic DC include UV irradiation, as well as exposure to CTLA-4Ig, TGF-beta or IL-10.[224-226] How a tolerogenic DC acts to suppress immunoreactivity is not completely understood, but may involve the promotion of anergy of T-cells that come into contact with DC, a shift from TH1 to TH2-type responses, apoptosis of the autoreactive T-cells or the induction of regulatory cells including regulatory T-cells and NK-T cells.[223,227-231] With the aim of establishing a durable tolerogenic state in the recipient of an allogeneic transplant, myeloid DC have been genetically modified using adenoviral and retroviral vectors encoding CTLA-4Ig, TGF-beta and IL-10 in the mouse.[224-226] CTLA-4Ig-expressing DC significantly prolong allograft survival, can induce alloantigen-specific T cell hyporesponsiveness, and display enhanced survival in nonimmunosuppressed, allogeneic hosts.[225] The in vivo presentation of alloantigens by donor or recipient DC in the absence of costimulation along with local production of immunosuppressive molecules like TGF-beta, could likely promote the inhibition of anti-donor reactivity and promote tolerance induction without causing any major systemic immunosuppression. DC engineered to express vIL-10 following retroviral gene transfer produce high levels of vIL-10 in vitro, exhibit marked reduction in cell surface MHC and costimulatory molecule expression, decrease T cell allostimulation and promote the induction of T cell hyporesponsiveness.[224] Genetically-engineered DC may be used to prevent islet allograft rejection, since they are able to manipulate anti-donor and/or autoantigen immunoreactivity. If recent observations showing islet-specific molecule gene expression in peripheral lymphoid organs can be confirmed in antigen presenting cells[232] like bone marrow-derived dendritic cells (Machen et al manuscript submitted), one can envision infusing autologous DC engineered ex vivo to lack costimulatory capability, but also express islet-specific genes (e.g., GAD65 or insulin), into prediabetic or early-onset diabetic patients, with the objective of inducing autoantigen-specific hyporesponsiveness. In fact, DC have been treated ex vivo with oligodeoxyribonucleotide decoys to NF-kB, an important maturational transcriptional mediator in DC, and injected into an allogeneic host. These DC were able to prolong the survival of an allogeneic heart.[233] It is likely that this and other transcriptional pathways in APC could be exploited by decoy nucleotide strategies to present autoantigen in the absence of costimulatory signals or in the presence of death ligands to silence or kill autoreactive T-cells.

Conclusion

While pharmacologic agents will no doubt continue to be discovered to promote safer immunosuppression, insulin sensitisation and enhancement of insulin output, diabetes mellitus will continue to be a challenging disorder in which these agents could be applied. Gene therapeutics, however, will take advantage of the knowledge of the underlying stage and severity of diabetes and will very likely be patient-specific. Nonetheless, a targeted approach, which is offered by gene medicines, is certainly much better than the systemic effects and toxicities that many drugs in use today are associated with.

References

1. Eisenbarth GS. Molecular aspects of the etiology of type I diabetes mellitus. J Diabetes Complications 1993; 7(2):142-150.
2. Bach JF. Insulin-dependent diabetes mellitus as an autoimmune disease. Endocr Rev 1994; 15(4):516-542.
3. Makino S, Kunimoto K, Muraoka Y et al. Breeding of a nonobese, diabetic strain of mice. Jikken Dobutsu 1980; 29(1):1-13.
4. Arreaza GA, Cameron MJ, Jaramillo A et al. Neonatal activation of CD28 signaling overcomes T cell anergy and prevents autoimmune diabetes by an IL-4-dependent mechanism. J Clin Invest 1997; 100(9):2243-2253.
5. Tiedge M, Lortz S, Munday R et al. Complementary action of antioxidant enzymes in the protection of bioengineered insulin-producing RINm5F cells against the toxicity of reactive oxygen species. Diabetes 1998; 47(10):1578-1585.
6. Markees TG, Serreze DV, Phillips NE et al. NOD mice have a generalized defect in their response to transplantation tolerance induction. Diabetes 1999; 48(5):967-974.
7. Leijon K, Hammarstrom B, Holmberg D. Nonobese diabetic (NOD) mice display enhanced immune responses and prolonged survival of lymphoid cells. Int Immunol 1994; 6(2):339-345.
8. Christianson SW, Shultz LD, Leiter EH. Adoptive transfer of diabetes into immunodeficient NOD-scid/scid mice. Relative contributions of CD4+ and CD8+ T-cells from diabetic versus prediabetic NOD.NONThy-1a donors. Diabetes 1993; 42(1):44-55.
9. Haskins K, McDuffie M. Acceleration of diabetes in young NOD mice with a CD4+ islet-specific T cell clone. Science 1990; 249(4975):1433-1436.
10. Miller BJ, Appel MC, O'Neil JJ et al. Both the Lyt-2+ and L3T4+ T cell subsets are required for the transfer of diabetes in nonobese diabetic mice. J Immunol 1988; 140(1):52-58.
11. O'Reilly LA, Hutchings PR, Crocker PR et al. Characterization of pancreatic islet cell infiltrates in NOD mice: Effect of cell transfer and transgene expression. Eur J Immunol 1991; 21(5):1171-1180.
12. DiLorenzo TP, Graser RT, Ono T et al. Major histocompatibility complex class I-restricted T cells are required for all but the end stages of diabetes development in nonobese diabetic mice and use a prevalent T cell receptor alpha chain gene rearrangement. Proc Natl Acad Sci USA 1998; 95(21):12538-12543.

13. Serreze DV, Chapman HD, Varnum DS et al. Initiation of autoimmune diabetes in NOD/Lt mice is MHC class I- dependent. J Immunol 1997; 158(8):3978-3986.
14. Graser RT, DiLorenzo TP, Wang F et al. Identification of a CD8 T cell that can independently mediate autoimmune diabetes development in the complete absence of CD4 T cell helper functions. J Immunol 2000; 164(7):3913-3918.
15. Katz JD, Wang B, Haskins K et al. Following a diabetogenic T cell from genesis through pathogenesis. Cell 1993; 74(6):1089-1100.
16. Eizirik DL, Flodstrom M, Karlsen AE et al. The harmony of the spheres: Inducible nitric oxide synthase and related genes in pancreatic beta cells. Diabetologia 1996; 39(8):875-890.
17. Mandrup-Poulsen T. The role of interleukin-1 in the pathogenesis of IDDM. Diabetologia 1996; 39(9):1005-1029.
18. Rabinovitch A, Suarez-Pinzon WL, Sorensen O et al. Inducible nitric oxide synthase (iNOS) in pancreatic islets of nonobese diabetic mice: Identification of iNOS- expressing cells and relationships to cytokines expressed in the islets. Endocrinology 1996; 137(5):2093-2099.
19. Corbett JA, Wang JL, Sweetland MA et al. Interleukin 1 beta induces the formation of nitric oxide by beta-cells purified from rodent islets of Langerhans. Evidence for the beta-cell as a source and site of action of nitric oxide. J Clin Invest 1992; 90(6):2384-2391.
20. Grankvist K, Marklund S, Sehlin J et al. Superoxide dismutase, catalase and scavengers of hydroxyl radical protect against the toxic action of alloxan on pancreatic islet cells in vitro. Biochem J 1979; 182(1):17-25.
21. Kroncke KD, Kolb-Bachofen V, Berschick B et al. Activated macrophages kill pancreatic syngeneic islet cells via arginine-dependent nitric oxide generation. Biochem Biophys Res Commun 1991; 175(3):752-758.
22. Lortz S, Tiedge M, Nachtwey T et al. Protection of insulin-producing RINm5F cells against cytokine-mediated toxicity through overexpression of antioxidant enzymes. Diabetes 2000; 49(7):1123-1130.
23. Chervonsky AV, Wang Y, Wong FS et al. The role of Fas in autoimmune diabetes. Cell 1997; 89(1):17-24.
24. Itoh N, Imagawa A, Hanafusa T et al. Requirement of Fas for the development of autoimmune diabetes in nonobese diabetic mice. J Exp Med 1997; 186(4):613-618.
25. Kaneto H, Fujii J, Seo HG et al. Apoptotic cell death triggered by nitric oxide in pancreatic beta-cells. Diabetes 1995; 44(7):733-738.
26. Kurrer MO, Pakala SV, Hanson HL et al. Beta cell apoptosis in T cell-mediated autoimmune diabetes. Proc Natl Acad Sci USA 1997; 94(1):213-218.
27. O'Brien BA, Harmon BV, Cameron DP et al. Apoptosis is the mode of beta-cell death responsible for the development of IDDM in the nonobese diabetic (NOD) mouse. Diabetes 1997; 46(5):750-757.
28. Benhamou PY, Moriscot C, Badet L et al. Strategies for graft immunomodulation in islet transplantation. Diabetes Metab 1998; 24(3):215-224.
29. Hohmeier HE, Thigpen A, Tran VV et al. Stable expression of manganese superoxide dismutase (MnSOD) in insulinoma cells prevents IL-1beta- induced cytotoxicity and reduces nitric oxide production. J Clin Invest 1998; 101(9):1811-1820.
30. Bertera S, Crawford ML, Alexander AM et al. Gene transfer of manganese superoxide dismutase extends islet graft function in a mouse model of autoimmune diabetes. Diabetes Feb 2003; 52(2):387-393.
31. Hotta M, Tashiro F, Ikegami H et al. Pancreatic beta cell-specific expression of thioredoxin, an antioxidative and antiapoptotic protein, prevents autoimmune and streptozotocin-induced diabetes. J Exp Med 1998; 188(8):1445-1451.
32. Kubisch HM, Wang J, Luche R et al. Transgenic copper/zinc superoxide dismutase modulates susceptibility to type I diabetes. Proc Natl Acad Sci USA 1994; 91(21):9956-9959.
33. Kubisch HM, Wang J, Bray TM et al. Targeted overexpression of Cu/Zn superoxide dismutase protects pancreatic beta-cells against oxidative stress. Diabetes 1997; 46(10):1563-1566.
34. Piganelli JD, Flores SC, Cruz C et al. A metalloporphyrin-based superoxide dismutase mimic inhibits adoptive transfer of autoimmune diabetes by a diabetogenic T-cell clone. Diabetes 2002; 51(2):347-355.

35. Bottino R, Balamurugan AN, Bertera S et al. Preservation of human islet cell functional mass by anti-oxidative action of a novel SOD mimic compound. Diabetes 2002; 51(8):2561-2567.
36. Wicker LS, Todd JA, Peterson LB. Genetic control of autoimmune diabetes in the NOD mouse. Annu Rev Immunol 1995; 13:179-200.
37. Vyse TJ, Todd JA. Genetic analysis of autoimmune disease. Cell 1996; 85(3):311-318.
38. Cordell HJ, Todd JA. Multifactorial inheritance in type 1 diabetes. Trends Genet 1995; 11(12):499-504.
39. Pietropaolo M, Becker DJ, LaPorte RE et al. Progression to insulin-requiring diabetes in seronegative prediabetic subjects: The role of two HLA-DQ high-risk haplotypes. Diabetologia 2002; 45(1):66-76.
40. Pietropaolo M, Trucco M. Major histocompatibility locus and other genes that determine risk of development of insulin-dependent diabetes mellitus. In: LeRoith D, Taylor S, Olefsky JM, eds. Diabetes Mellitus: A fundamental and Clinical Text. 2nd ed. Philadelphia, PA: J.B. Lippincott & Co., 2000:399-410.
41. Vafiadis P, Bennett ST, Todd JA et al. Insulin expression in human thymus is modulated by INS VNTR alleles at the IDDM2 locus. Nat Genet 1997; 15(3):289-292.
42. Pugliese A, Zeller M, Fernandez Jr A et al. The insulin gene is transcribed in the human thymus and transcription levels correlated with allelic variation at the INS VNTR-IDDM2 susceptibility locus for type 1 diabetes. Nat Genet 1997; 15(3):293-297.
43. Chentoufi AA, Polychronakos C. Insulin expression levels in the thymus modulate insulin-specific autoreactive T-cell tolerance: The mechanism by which the IDDM2 locus may predispose to diabetes. Diabetes 2002; 51(5):1383-1390.
44. Mein CA, Esposito L, Dunn MG et al. A search for type 1 diabetes susceptibility genes in families from the United Kingdom. Nat Genet 1998; 19(3):297-300.
45. Concannon P, Gogolin-Ewens KJ, Hinds DA et al. A second-generation screen of the human genome for susceptibility to insulin-dependent diabetes mellitus. Nat Genet 1998; 19(3):292-296.
46. Davies JL, Kawaguchi Y, Bennett ST et al. A genome-wide search for human type 1 diabetes susceptibility genes. Nature 1994; 371(6493):130-136.
47. Oldstone MB. Molecular mimicry and immune-mediated diseases. Faseb J 1998; 12(13):1255-1265.
48. von Herrath MG, Holz A, Homann D et al. Role of viruses in type I diabetes. Semin Immunol 1998; 10(1):87-100.
49. Horwitz MS, Bradley LM, Harbertson J et al. Diabetes induced by Coxsackie virus: Initiation by bystander damage and not molecular mimicry. Nat Med 1998; 4(7):781-785.
50. Karges W, Hammond-McKibben D, Cheung RK et al. Immunological aspects of nutritional diabetes prevention in NOD mice: A pilot study for the cow's milk-based IDDM prevention trial. Diabetes 1997; 46(4):557-564.
51. Kaufman DL, Erlander MG, ClareSalzler M et al. Autoimmunity to two forms of glutamate decarboxylase in insulin- dependent diabetes mellitus. J Clin Invest 1992; 89(1):283-292.
52. Conrad B, Trucco M. Superantigens as etiopathogenetic factors in the development of insulin-dependent diabetes mellitus. Diabetes Metab Rev 1994; 10(4):309-338.
53. Conrad B, Weidmann E, Trucco G et al. Evidence for superantigen involvement in insulin-dependent diabetes mellitus aetiology. Nature 1994; 371(6495):351-355.
54. Acerini CL, Ahmed ML, Ross KM et al. Coeliac disease in children and adolescents with IDDM: Clinical characteristics and response to gluten-free diet. Diabet Med 1998; 15(1):38-44.
55. Virtanen SM, Saukkonen T, Savilahti E et al. Diet, cow's milk protein antibodies and the risk of IDDM in Finnish children. Childhood Diabetes in Finland Study Group. Diabetologia 1994; 37(4):381-387.
56. Kostraba JN, Dorman JS, LaPorte RE et al. Early infant diet and risk of IDDM in blacks and whites. A matched case- control study. Diabetes Care 1992; 15(5):626-631.
57. Berney T, Buhler L, Caulfield A et al. Transplantation of islets of Langerhans: New developments. Swiss Med Wkly 2001; 131(47-48):671-680.
58. Boker A, Rothenberg L, Hernandez C et al. Human islet transplantation: Update. World J Surg 2001; 25(4):481-486.
59. Berney T, Ricordi C. Islet cell transplantation: The future? Langenbecks Arch Surg 2000; 385(6):373-378.

60. Berney T, Ricordi C. Islet transplantation. Cell Transplant 1999; 8(5):461-464.
61. Shapiro AM, Lakey JR, Ryan EA et al. Islet transplantation in seven patients with type 1 diabetes mellitus using a glucocorticoid-free immunosuppressive regimen. N Engl J Med 2000; 343(4):230-238.
62. Ryan EA, Lakey JR, Shapiro AM. Clinical results after islet transplantation. J Investig Med 2001; 49(6):559-562.
63. Shapiro AM, Ryan EA, Lakey JR. Pancreatic islet transplantation in the treatment of diabetes mellitus. Best Pract Res Clin Endocrinol Metab 2001; 15(2):241-264.
64. Ryan EA, Lakey JR, Rajotte RV et al. Clinical outcomes and insulin secretion after islet transplantation with the Edmonton protocol. Diabetes 2001; 50(4):710-719.
65. Bottino R, Trucco M, Balamurugan AN et al. Pancreas and islet cell transplantation. Best Pract Res Clin Gastroenterol 2002; 16(3):457-474.
66. Jaeschke H. Vascular oxidant stress and hepatic ischemia/reperfusion injury. Free Radic Res Commun 1991; 12-13(Pt 2):737-743.
67. Jaeschke H. Reactive oxygen and ischemia/reperfusion injury of the liver. Chem Biol Interact 1991; 79(2):115-136.
68. Paraskevas S, Maysinger D, Wang R et al. Cell loss in isolated human islets occurs by apoptosis. Pancreas 2000; 20(3):270-276.
69. Rosenberg L, Wang R, Paraskevas S et al. Structural and functional changes resulting from islet isolation lead to islet cell death. Surgery 1999; 126(2):393-398.
70. Nagano H, Tilney NL. Chronic allograft failure: The clinical problem. Am J Med Sci 1997; 313(5):305-309.
71. Bulkley GB. Free radical-mediated reperfusion injury: A selective review. Br J Cancer Suppl 1987; 8:66-73.
72. Pileggi A, Molano RD, Berney T et al. Heme oxygenase-1 induction in islet cells results in protection from apoptosis and improved in vivo function after transplantation. Diabetes 2001; 50(9):1983-1991.
73. Tobiasch E, Gunther L, Bach FH. Heme oxygenase-1 protects pancreatic beta cells from apoptosis caused by various stimuli. J Investig Med 2001; 49(6):566-571.
74. Contreras JL, Bilbao G, Smyth C et al. Gene transfer of the Bcl-2 gene confers cytoprotection to isolated adult porcine pancreatic islets exposed to xenoreactive antibodies and complement. Surgery 2001; 130(2):166-174.
75. Contreras JL, Bilbao G, Smyth CA et al. Cytoprotection of pancreatic islets before and soon after transplantation by gene transfer of the anti-apoptotic Bcl-2 gene. Transplantation 2001; 71(8):1015-1023.
76. Lortz S, Tiedge M, Nachtwey T et al. Protection of insulin-producing RINm5F cells against cytokine-mediated toxicity through overexpression of antioxidant enzymes. Diabetes 2000; 49(7):1123-1130.
77. Hotta M, Tashiro F, Ikegami H et al. Pancreatic beta cell-specific expression of thioredoxin, an antioxidative and antiapoptotic protein, prevents autoimmune and streptozotocin-induced diabetes. J Exp Med 1998; 188(8):1445-1451.
78. Embury J, Klein D, Pileggi A et al. Proteins linked to a protein transduction domain efficiently transduce pancreatic islets. Diabetes 2001; 50(8):1706-1713.
79. Jaeschke H, Smith CW, Clemens MG et al. Mechanisms of inflammatory liver injury: Adhesion molecules and cytotoxicity of neutrophils. Toxicol Appl Pharmacol 1996; 139(2):213-226.
80. Jaeschke H. Chemokines, neutrophils, and inflammatory liver injury. Shock 1996; 6(6):403-404.
81. Dairaghi DJ, Fan RA, McMaster BE et al. HHV8-encoded vMIP-I selectively engages chemokine receptor CCR8. Agonist and antagonist profiles of viral chemokines. J Biol Chem 1999; 274(31):21569-21574.
82. Howard OM, Oppenheim JJ, Wang JM. Chemokines as molecular targets for therapeutic intervention. J Clin Immunol 1999; 19(5):280-292.
83. Dong H, Woo SL. Hepatic insulin production for type 1 diabetes. Trends Endocrinol Metab 2001; 12(10):441-446.
84. Dong H, Morral N, McEvoy R et al. Hepatic insulin expression improves glycemic control in type 1 diabetic rats. Diabetes Res Clin Pract 2001; 52(3):153-163.

85. Thule PM, Liu JM. Regulated hepatic insulin gene therapy of STZ-diabetic rats. Gene Ther 2000; 7(20):1744-1752.
86. Mitanchez D, Rabier D, Mokhtari M et al. 5-Oxoprolinuria: A cause of neonatal metabolic acidosis. Acta Paediatr 2001; 90(7):827-828.
87. Mitanchez D, Chen R, Massias JF et al. Regulated expression of mature human insulin in the liver of transgenic mice. FEBS Lett 1998; 421(3):285-289.
88. Mitanchez D, Doiron B, Chen R et al. Glucose-stimulated genes and prospects of gene therapy for type I diabetes. Endocr Rev 1997; 18(4):520-540.
89. Flotte T, Agarwal A, Wang J et al. Efficient ex vivo transduction of pancreatic islet cells with recombinant adeno-associated virus vectors. Diabetes 2001; 50(3):515-520.
90. Lee HC, Kim SJ, Kim KS et al. Remission in models of type 1 diabetes by gene therapy using a single- chain insulin analogue. Nature 2000; 408(6811):483-488.
91. Yang YW, Kotin RM. Glucose-responsive gene delivery in pancreatic Islet cells via recombinant adeno-associated viral vectors. Pharm Res 2000; 17(9):1056-1061.
92. Yang YW, Hsieh YC. Regulated secretion of proinsulin/insulin from human hepatoma cells transduced by recombinant adeno-associated virus. Biotechnol Appl Biochem 2001; 33(Pt 2):133-140.
93. Bochan MR, Sidner RA, Shah R et al. Stable transduction of human pancreatic adenocarcinoma cells, rat fibroblasts, and bone marrow-derived stem cells with recombinant adeno- associated virus containing the rat preproinsulin II gene. Transplant Proc 1998; 30(2):453-454.
94. Kasten-Jolly J, Aubrey MT, Conti DJ et al. Reversal of hyperglycemia in diabetic NOD mice by human proinsulin gene therapy. Transplant Proc 1997; 29(4):2216-2218.
95. Bartlett RJ, Denis M, Secore SL et al. Toward engineering skeletal muscle to release peptide hormone from the human preproinsulin gene. Transplant Proc 1998; 30(2):451.
96. Simpson AM, Marshall GM, Tuch BE et al. Gene therapy of diabetes: Glucose-stimulated insulin secretion in a human hepatoma cell line (HEP G2ins/g). Gene Ther 1997; 4(11):1202-1215.
97. Simonson GD, Groskreutz DJ, Gorman CM et al. Synthesis and processing of genetically modified human proinsulin by rat myoblast primary cultures. Hum Gene Ther 1996; 7(1):71-78.
98. Rajagopal J, Anderson WJ, Kume S et al. Insulin staining of ES cell progeny from insulin uptake. Science Jan 17 2003; 299(5605):363.
99. Vollenweider F, Irminger JC, Halban PA. Substrate specificity of proinsulin conversion in the constitutive pathway of transfected FAO (hepatoma) cells. Diabetologia 1993; 36(12):1322-1325.
100. Vollenweider F, Irminger JC, Gross DJ et al. Processing of proinsulin by transfected hepatoma (FAO) cells. J Biol Chem 1992; 267(21):14629-14636.
101. Groskreutz DJ, Sliwkowski MX, Gorman CM. Genetically engineered proinsulin constitutively processed and secreted as mature, active insulin. J Biol Chem 1994; 269(8):6241-6245.
102. Mitanchez D, Chen R, Massias JF et al. Regulated expression of mature human insulin in the liver of transgenic mice. FEBS Lett 1998; 421(3):285-289.
103. Mitanchez D, Doiron B, Chen R et al. Glucose-stimulated genes and prospects of gene therapy for type I diabetes. Endocr Rev 1997; 18(4):520-540.
104. Thule PM, Liu J, Phillips LS. Glucose regulated production of human insulin in rat hepatocytes. Gene Ther 2000; 7(3):205-214.
105. Chen R, Meseck ML, Woo SL. Auto-regulated hepatic insulin gene expression in type 1 diabetic rats. Mol Ther 2001; 3(4):584-590.
106. Chen R, Meseck M, McEvoy RC et al. Glucose-stimulated and self-limiting insulin production by glucose 6- phosphatase promoter driven insulin expression in hepatoma cells. Gene Ther 2000; 7(21):1802-1809.
107. Iynedjian PB, Jotterand D, Nouspikel T et al. Transcriptional induction of glucokinase gene by insulin in cultured liver cells and its repression by the glucagon-cAMP system. J Biol Chem 1989; 264(36):21824-21829.
108. Iynedjian PB, Pilot PR, Nouspikel T et al. Differential expression and regulation of the glucokinase gene in liver and islets of Langerhans. Proc Natl Acad Sci USA 1989; 86(20):7838-7842.
109. Liu JS, Park EA, Gurney AL et al. Cyclic AMP induction of phosphoenolpyruvate carboxykinase (GTP) gene transcription is mediated by multiple promoter elements. J Biol Chem 1991; 266(28):19095-19102.

110. Klemm DJ, Roesler WJ, Liu JS et al. In vitro analysis of promoter elements regulating transcription of the phosphoenolpyruvate carboxykinase (GTP) gene. Mol Cell Biol 1990; 10(2):480-485.
111. Lipes MA, Cooper EM, Skelly R et al. Insulin-secreting nonislet cells are resistant to autoimmune destruction. Proc Natl Acad Sci USA 1996; 93(16):8595-8600.
112. Lipes MA, Davalli AM, Cooper EM. Genetic engineering of insulin expression in nonislet cells: Implications for beta-cell replacement therapy for insulin-dependent diabetes mellitus. Acta Diabetol 1997; 34(1):2-5.
113. Cheung AT, Dayanandan B, Lewis JT et al. Glucose-dependent insulin release from genetically engineered K cells. Science 2000; 290(5498):1959-1962.
114. Cornelius JG, Tchernev V, Kao KJ et al. In vitro-generation of islets in long-term cultures of pluripotent stem cells from adult mouse pancreas. Horm Metab Res 1997; 29(6):271-277.
115. Beattie GM, Rubin JS, Mally MI et al. Regulation of proliferation and differentiation of human fetal pancreatic islet cells by extracellular matrix, hepatocyte growth factor, and cell-cell contact. Diabetes 1996; 45(9):1223-1228.
116. Beattie GM, Lopez AD, Hayek A. In vivo maturation and growth potential of human fetal pancreases: Fresh versus cultured tissue. Transplant Proc 1995; 27(6):3343.
117. Beattie GM, Hayek A. Outcome of human fetal pancreatic transplants according to implantation site. Transplant Proc 1994; 26(6):3299.
118. Beattie GM, Cirulli V, Lopez AD et al. Ex vivo expansion of human pancreatic endocrine cells. J Clin Endocrinol Metab 1997; 82(6):1852-1856.
119. Lumelsky N, Blondel O, Laeng P et al. Differentiation of embryonic stem cells to insulin-secreting structures similar to pancreatic islets. Science 2001; 292(5520):1389-1394.
120. Wagers AJ, Christensen JL, Weissman IL. Cell fate determination from stem cells. Gene Ther 2002; 9(10):606-612.
121. McKay R. Stem cells—hype and hope. Nature 2000; 406(6794):361-364.
122. Jiang Y, Jahagirdar BN, Reinhardt RL et al. Pluripotency of mesenchymal stem cells derived from adult marrow. Nature 2002; 418(6893):41-49.
123. Schwartz RE, Reyes M, Koodie L et al. Multipotent adult progenitor cells from bone marrow differentiate into functional hepatocyte-like cells. J Clin Invest 2002; 109(10):1291-1302.
124. Reyes M, Verfaillie CM. Characterization of multipotent adult progenitor cells, a subpopulation of mesenchymal stem cells. Ann N Y Acad Sci 2001; 938:231-233 discussion 233-235.
125. Colman A, Kind A. Therapeutic cloning: Concepts and practicalities. Trends Biotechnol 2000; 18(5):192-196.
126. Kind A, Colman A. Therapeutic cloning: Needs and prospects. Semin Cell Dev Biol 1999; 10(3):279-286.
127. Lanza RP, Cibelli JB, West MD. Human therapeutic cloning. Nat Med 1999; 5(9):975-977.
128. D'Ambra R, Surana M, Efrat S et al. Regulation of insulin secretion from beta-cell lines derived from transgenic mice insulinomas resembles that of normal beta-cells. Endocrinology 1990; 126(6):2815-2822.
129. Efrat S, Fusco-DeMane D, Lemberg H et al. Conditional transformation of a pancreatic beta-cell line derived from transgenic mice expressing a tetracycline-regulated oncogene. Proc Natl Acad Sci USA 1995; 92(8):3576-3580.
130. Efrat S. Cell-based therapy for insulin-dependent diabetes mellitus. Eur J Endocrinol 1998; 138(2):129-133.
131. Fleischer N, Chen C, Surana M et al. Functional analysis of a conditionally transformed pancreatic beta-cell line. Diabetes 1998; 47(9):1419-1425.
132. Hayek A, Beattie GM, Cirulli V et al. Growth factor/matrix-induced proliferation of human adult beta-cells. Diabetes 1995; 44(12):1458-1460.
133. Otonkoski T, Beattie GM, Rubin JS et al. Hepatocyte growth factor/scatter factor has insulinotropic activity in human fetal pancreatic cells. Diabetes 1994; 43(7):947-953.
134. Otonkoski T, Cirulli V, Beattie M et al. A role for hepatocyte growth factor/scatter factor in fetal mesenchyme- induced pancreatic beta-cell growth. Endocrinology 1996; 137(7):3131-3139.
135. Levine F, Leibowitz G. Towards gene therapy of diabetes mellitus. Mol Med Today 1999; 5(4):165-171.

136. Beattie GM, Itkin-Ansari P, Cirulli V et al. Sustained proliferation of PDX-1+ cells derived from human islets. Diabetes 1999; 48(5):1013-1019.
137. Habener JF, Stoffers DA. A newly discovered role of transcription factors involved in pancreas development and the pathogenesis of diabetes mellitus. Proc Assoc Am Physicians 1998; 110(1):12-21.
138. Madsen OD, Jensen J, Petersen HV et al. Transcription factors contributing to the pancreatic beta-cell phenotype. Horm Metab Res 1997; 29(6):265-270.
139. Sander M, German MS. The beta cell transcription factors and development of the pancreas. J Mol Med 1997; 75(5):327-340.
140. Ferber S, Halkin A, Cohen H et al. Pancreatic and duodenal homeobox gene 1 induces expression of insulin genes in liver and ameliorates streptozotocin-induced hyperglycemia. Nat Med 2000; 6(5):568-572.
141. Wu KL, Gannon M, Peshavaria M et al. Hepatocyte nuclear factor 3beta is involved in pancreatic beta-cell- specific transcription of the pdx-1 gene. Mol Cell Biol 1997; 17(10):6002-6013.
142. Sander M, German MS. The beta cell transcription factors and development of the pancreas. J Mol Med 1997; 75(5):327-340.
143. Oster A, Jensen J, Serup P et al. Rat endocrine pancreatic development in relation to two homeobox gene products (Pdx-1 and Nkx 6.1). J Histochem Cytochem 1998; 46(6):707-715.
144. Hill DJ, Hogg J. Growth factor control of pancreatic B cell hyperplasia. Baillieres Clin Endocrinol Metab 1991; 5(4):689-698.
145. Ilieva A, Yuan S, Wang RN et al. Pancreatic islet cell survival following islet isolation: The role of cellular interactions in the pancreas. J Endocrinol 1999; 161(3):357-364.
146. Miettinen PJ, Otonkoski T, Voutilainen R. Insulin-like growth factor-II and transforming growth factor-alpha in developing human fetal pancreatic.islets. J Endocrinol 1993; 138(1):127-136.
147. Petrik J, Arany E, McDonald TJ et al. Apoptosis in the pancreatic islet cells of the neonatal rat is associated with a reduced expression of insulin-like growth factor II that may act as a survival factor. Endocrinology 1998; 139(6):2994-3004.
148. Petrik J, Pell JM, Arany E et al. Overexpression of insulin-like growth factor-II in transgenic mice is associated with pancreatic islet cell hyperplasia. Endocrinology 1999; 140(5):2353-2363.
149. Markoff E, Beattie GM, Hayek A et al. Effects of prolactin and glycosylated prolactin on (pro)insulin synthesis and insulin release from cultured rat pancreatic islets. Pancreas 1990; 5(1):99-103.
150. Kawai M, Kishi K. In vitro studies of the stimulation of insulin secretion and B-cell proliferation by rat placental lactogen-II during pregnancy in rats. J Reprod Fertil 1997; 109(1):145-152.
151. Billestrup N, Nielsen JH. The stimulatory effect of growth hormone, prolactin, and placental lactogen on beta-cell proliferation is not mediated by insulin-like growth factor-I. Endocrinology 1991; 129(2):883-888.
152. Vasavada RC, Cavaliere C, D'Ercole AJ et al. Overexpression of parathyroid hormone-related protein in the pancreatic islets of transgenic mice causes islet hyperplasia, hyperinsulinemia, and hypoglycemia. J Biol Chem 1996; 271(2):1200-1208.
153. Porter SE, Sorenson RL, Dann P et al. Progressive pancreatic islet hyperplasia in the islet-targeted, parathyroid hormone-related protein-overexpressing mouse. Endocrinology 1998; 139(9):3743-3751.
154. Wang RN, Rehfeld JF, Nielsen FC et al. Expression of gastrin and transforming growth factor-alpha during duct to islet cell differentiation in the pancreas of duct-ligated adult rats. Diabetologia 1997; 40(8):887-893.
155. Miettinen PJ, Otonkoski T, Voutilainen R. Insulin-like growth factor-II and transforming growth factor-alpha in developing human fetal pancreatic islets. J Endocrinol 1993; 138(1):127-136.
156. Miettinen PJ. Transforming growth factor-alpha and epidermal growth factor expression in human fetal gastrointestinal tract. Pediatr Res 1993; 33(5):481-486.
157. Baeza N, Hart A, Ahlgren U et al. Insulin promoter factor-1 controls several aspects of beta-cell identity. Diabetes 2001; 50 Suppl 1:S36.
158. Hart AW, Baeza N, Apelqvist A et al. Attenuation of FGF signalling in mouse beta-cells leads to diabetes. Nature 2000; 408(6814):864-868.
159. Yamaoka T, Itakura M. Development of pancreatic islets (review). Int J Mol Med 1999; 3(3):247-261.

160. Mally MI, Otonkoski T, Lopez AD et al. Developmental gene expression in the human fetal pancreas. Pediatr Res 1994; 36(4):537-544.
161. Unno M, Itoh T, Watanabe T et al. Islet beta-cell regeneration and reg genes. Adv Exp Med Biol 1992; 321:61-66.
162. Zenilman ME, Chen J, Danesh B et al. Characteristics of rat pancreatic regenerating protein. Surgery 1998; 124(5):855-863.
163. Zenilman ME, Chen J, Magnuson TH. Effect of reg protein on rat pancreatic ductal cells. Pancreas 1998; 17(3):256-261.
164. Bone AJ, Banister SH, Zhang S. The REG gene and islet cell repair and renewal in type 1 diabetes. Adv Exp Med Biol 1997; 426:321-327.
165. Vinik A, Rafaeloff R, Pittenger G et al. Induction of pancreatic islet neogenesis. Horm Metab Res 1997; 29(6):278-293.
166. Rafaeloff R, Pittenger GL, Barlow SW et al. Cloning and sequencing of the pancreatic islet neogenesis associated protein (INGAP) gene and its expression in islet neogenesis in hamsters. J Clin Invest 1997; 99(9):2100-2109.
167. Bonner-Weir S, Taneja M, Weir GC et al. In vitro cultivation of human islets from expanded ductal tissue. Proc Natl Acad Sci USA 2000; 97(14):7999-8004.
168. Dai Y, Vaught TD, Boone J et al. Targeted disruption of the alpha1,3-galactosyltransferase gene in cloned pigs. Nat Biotechnol 2002; 20(3):251-255.
169. Koike C, Fung JJ, Geller DA et al. Molecular basis of evolutionary loss of the alpha 1,3-galactosyltransferase gene in higher primates. J Biol Chem 2002; 277(12):10114-10120.
170. Phelps CJ, Koike C, Vaught TD et al. Production of {alpha}1,3-Galactosyltransferase-Deficient Pigs. Science 2002; 19:19.
171. Giannoukakis N, Rudert WA, Robbins PD et al. Targeting autoimmune diabetes with gene therapy. Diabetes 1999; 48(11):2107-2121.
172. Giannoukakis N, Thomson A, Robbins P. Gene therapy in transplantation. Gene Ther 1999; 6(9):1499-1511.
173. Sui G, Soohoo C, Affar el B et al. A DNA vector-based RNAi technology to suppress gene expression in mammalian cells. Proc Natl Acad Sci USA 2002; 99(8):5515-5520.
174. Kogure K, Urabe M, Mizukami H et al. Targeted integration of foreign DNA into a defined locus on chromosome 19 in K562 cells using AAV-derived components. Int J Hematol 2001; 73(4):469-475.
175. Pieroni L, Fipaldini C, Monciotti A et al. Targeted integration of adeno-associated virus-derived plasmids in transfected human cells. Virology 1998; 249(2):249-259.
176. Ikeda Y, Collins MK, Radcliffe PA et al. Gene transduction efficiency in cells of different species by HIV and EIAV vectors. Gene Ther 2002; 9(14):932-938.
177. O'Rourke JP, Newbound GC, Kohn DB et al. Comparison of gene transfer efficiencies and gene expression levels achieved with equine infectious anemia virus- and human immunodeficiency virus type 1-derived lentivirus vectors. J Virol 2002; 76(3):1510-1515.
178. Olsen JC. Gene transfer vectors derived from equine infectious anemia virus. Gene Ther 1998; 5(11):1481-1487.
179. Lotery AJ, Derksen TA, Russell SR et al. Gene transfer to the nonhuman primate retina with recombinant feline immunodeficiency virus vectors. Hum Gene Ther 2002; 13(6):689-696.
180. Kelly PF, Vandergriff J, Nathwani A et al. Highly efficient gene transfer into cord blood nonobese diabetic/severe combined immunodeficiency repopulating cells by oncoretroviral vector particles pseudotyped with the feline endogenous retrovirus (RD114) envelope protein. Blood 2000; 96(4):1206-1214.
181. Curran MA, Kaiser SM, Achacoso PL et al. Efficient transduction of nondividing cells by optimized feline immunodeficiency virus vectors. Mol Ther 2000; 1(1):31-38.
182. Poeschla EM, Wong-Staal F, Looney DJ. Efficient transduction of nondividing human cells by feline immunodeficiency virus lentiviral vectors. Nat Med 1998; 4(3):354-357.
183. Britt LD, Scharp DW, Lacy PE et al. Transplantation of islet cells across major histocompatibility barriers after total lymphoid irradiation and infusion of allogeneic bone marrow cells. Diabetes 1982; 31 Suppl 4:63-68.

184. Exner BG, Fowler K, Ildstad ST. Tolerance induction for islet transplantation. Ann Transplant 1997; 2(3):77-80.
185. Rossini AA, Parker DC, Phillips NE et al. Induction of immunological tolerance to islet allografts. Cell Transplant 1996; 5(1):49-52.
186. Domenick MA, Ildstad ST. Impact of bone marrow transplantation on type I diabetes. World J Surg 2001; 25(4):474-480.
187. Good RA, Verjee T. Historical and current perspectives on bone marrow transplantation for prevention and treatment of immunodeficiencies and autoimmunities. Biol Blood Marrow Transplant 2001; 7(3):123-135.
188. Mathieu C, Bouillon R, Rutgeerts O et al. Induction of mixed bone marrow chimerism as potential therapy for autoimmune (type I) diabetes: Experience in the NOD model. Transplant Proc 1995; 27(1):640-641.
189. Mathieu C, Vandeputte M, Bouillon R et al. Protection against autoimmune diabetes by induction of mixed bone marrow chimerism. Transplant Proc 1993; 25(1 Pt 2):1266-1267.
190. Li H, Kaufman CL, Ildstad ST. Allogeneic chimerism induces donor-specific tolerance to simultaneous islet allografts in nonobese diabetic mice. Surgery 1995; 118(2):192-197 discussion 197-198.
191. Li H, Inverardi L, Ricordi C. Chimerism-induced remission of overt diabetes in nonobese diabetic mice. Transplant Proc 1999; 31(1-2):640.
192. Zorina TD, Subbotin VM, Bertera S et al. Distinct characteristics and features of allogeneic chimerism in the NOD mouse model of autoimmune diabetes. Cell Transplant 2002; 11(2):113-123.
193. Feili-Hariri M, Dong X, Alber SM et al. Immunotherapy of NOD mice with bone marrow-derived dendritic cells. Diabetes 1999; 48(12):2300-2308.
194. Clare-Salzler MJ, Brooks J, Chai A et al. Prevention of diabetes in nonobese diabetic mice by dendritic cell transfer. J Clin Invest 1992; 90(3):741-748.
195. Giannoukakis N, Bonham CA, Qian S et al. Prolongation of cardiac allograft survival using dendritic cells treated with NF-kB decoy oligodeoxyribonucleotides. Mol Ther 2000; 1(5 Pt 1):430-437.
196. Lu L, Thomson AW. Manipulation of dendritic cells for tolerance induction in transplantation and autoimmune disease. Transplantation 2002; 73(1 Suppl):S19-22.
197. Lu L, Gambotto A, Lee WC et al. Adenoviral delivery of CTLA4Ig into myeloid dendritic cells promotes their in vitro tolerogenicity and survival in allogeneic recipients. Gene Ther 1999; 6(4):554-563.
198. Lu L, Lee WC, Takayama T et al. Genetic engineering of dendritic cells to express immunosuppressive molecules (viral IL-10, TGF-beta, and CTLA4Ig). J Leukoc Biol 1999; 66(2):293-296.
199. Thomson AW, Lu L. Dendritic cells as regulators of immune reactivity: Implications for transplantation. Transplantation 1999; 68(1):1-8.
200. Lee WC, Zhong C, Qian S et al. Phenotype, function, and in vivo migration and survival of allogeneic dendritic cell progenitors genetically engineered to express TGF-beta. Transplantation 1998; 66(12):1810-1817.
201. Takayama T, Nishioka Y, Lu L et al. Retroviral delivery of viral interleukin-10 into myeloid dendritic cells markedly inhibits their allostimulatory activity and promotes the induction of T-cell hyporesponsiveness. Transplantation 1998; 66(12):1567-1574.
202. Rosenbloom AL, Schatz DA, Krischer JP et al. Therapeutic controversy: Prevention and treatment of diabetes in children. J Clin Endocrinol Metab 2000; 85(2):494-522.
203. Wilson K, Eisenbarth GS. Immunopathogenesis and immunotherapy of type 1 diabetes. Annu Rev Med 1990; 41:497-508.
204. Papoz L, Lenegre F, Hors J et al. Probability of remission in individual in early adult insulin dependent diabetic patients. Results from the Cyclosporine Diabetes French Study Group. Diabete Metab 1990; 16(4):303-310.
205. Shimada A, Imazu Y, Morinaga S et al. T-cell insulitis found in anti-GAD65+ diabetes with residual beta-cell function. A case report. Diabetes Care 1999; 22(4):615-617.
206. Hamamoto Y, Tsuura Y, Fujimoto S et al. Recovery of function and mass of endogenous beta-cells in streptozotocin-induced diabetic rats treated with islet transplantation. Biochem Biophys Res Commun 2001; 287(1):104-109.

207. Rasmussen SB, Sorensen TS, Hansen JB et al. Functional rest through intensive treatment with insulin and potassium channel openers preserves residual beta-cell function and mass in acutely diabetic BB rats. Horm Metab Res 2000; 32(7):294-300.
208. Mayer A, Rharbaoui F, Thivolet C et al. The relationship between peripheral T cell reactivity to insulin, clinical remissions and cytokine production in type 1 (insulin- dependent) diabetes mellitus. J Clin Endocrinol Metab 1999; 84(7):2419-2424.
209. Finegood DT, Weir GC, Bonner-Weir S. Prior streptozotocin treatment does not inhibit pancreas regeneration after 90% pancreatectomy in rats. Am J Physiol 1999; 276(5 Pt 1):E822-827.
210. Chatenoud L, Thervet E, Primo J et al. Anti-CD3 antibody induces long-term remission of overt autoimmunity in nonobese diabetic mice. Proc Natl Acad Sci USA 1994; 91(1):123-127.
211. Herold KC, Hagopian W, Auger JA et al. Anti-CD3 monoclonal antibody in new-onset type 1 diabetes mellitus. N Engl J Med 2002; 346(22):1692-1698.
212. Arnush M, Heitmeier MR, Scarim AL et al. IL-1 produced and released endogenously within human islets inhibits beta cell function. J Clin Invest 1998; 102(3):516-526.
213. Arnush M, Scarim AL, Heitmeier MR et al. Potential role of resident islet macrophage activation in the initiation of autoimmune diabetes. J Immunol 1998; 160(6):2684-2691.
214. Corbett JA, McDaniel ML. Intraislet release of interleukin 1 inhibits beta cell function by inducing beta cell expression of inducible nitric oxide synthase. J Exp Med 1995; 181(2):559-568.
215. Heitmeier MR, Scarim AL, Corbett JA. Interferon-gamma increases the sensitivity of islets of Langerhans for inducible nitric-oxide synthase expression induced by interleukin 1. J Biol Chem 1997; 272(21):13697-13704.
216. Lacy PE. The intraislet macrophage and type I diabetes. Mt Sinai J Med 1994; 61(2):170-174.
217. McDaniel ML, Kwon G, Hill JR et al. Cytokines and nitric oxide in islet inflammation and diabetes. Proc Soc Exp Biol Med 1996; 211(1):24-32.
218. Scarim AL, Arnush M, Hill JR et al. Evidence for the presence of type I IL-1 receptors on beta-cells of islets of Langerhans. Biochim Biophys Acta 1997; 1361(3):313-320.
219. French MB, Allison J, Cram DS et al. Transgenic expression of mouse proinsulin II prevents diabetes in nonobese diabetic mice. Diabetes 1997; 46(1):34-39.
220. Miyazaki T, Matsuda Y, Toyonaga T et al. Prevention of autoimmune insulitis in nonobese diabetic mice by expression of major histocompatibility complex class I Ld molecules. Proc Natl Acad Sci USA 1992; 89(20):9519-9523.
221. Gerling IC, Serreze DV, Christianson SW et al. Intrathymic islet cell transplantation reduces beta-cell autoimmunity and prevents diabetes in NOD/Lt mice. Diabetes 1992; 41(12):1672-1676.
222. Leykin I, Nikolic B, Sykes M. Mixed bone marrow chimerism as a treatment for autoimmune diabetes. Transplant Proc 2001; 33(1-2):120.
223. Steptoe RJ, Thomson AW. Dendritic cells and tolerance induction. Clin Exp Immunol 1996; 105(3):397-402.
224. Takayama T, Nishioka Y, Lu L et al. Retroviral delivery of viral interleukin-10 into myeloid dendritic cells markedly inhibits their allostimulatory activity and promotes the induction of T-cell hyporesponsiveness. Transplantation 1998; 66(12):1567-1574.
225. Lu L, Lee WC, Gambotto A et al. Transduction of dendritic cells with adenoviral vectors encoding CTLA4-Ig markedly reduces their allostimulatory activity 1998.
226. Lee WC et al. Phenotype, function and in vivo migration and survival of allogeneic dendritic cell progenitors genetically engineered to express TGFb. Transplantation 1998 in press.
227. Sharif S, Arreaza GA, Zucker P et al. Regulatory natural killer T cells protect against spontaneous and recurrent type 1 diabetes. Ann N Y Acad Sci 2002; 958:77-88.
228. Naumov YN, Bahjat KS, Gausling R et al. Activation of CD1d-restricted T cells protects NOD mice from developing diabetes by regulating dendritic cell subsets. Proc Natl Acad Sci USA 2001; 98(24):13838-13843.
229. Sharif S, Delovitch TL. Regulation of immune responses by natural killer T cells. Arch Immunol Ther Exp (Warsz) 2001; 49(Suppl 1):S23-31.
230. Sharif S, Arreaza GA, Zucker P et al. Activation of natural killer T cells by alpha-galactosylceramide treatment prevents the onset and recurrence of autoimmune Type 1 diabetes. Nat Med 2001; 7(9):1057-1062.

231. Hong S, Wilson MT, Serizawa I et al. The natural killer T-cell ligand alpha-galactosylceramide prevents autoimmune diabetes in nonobese diabetic mice. Nat Med 2001; 7(9):1052-1056.
232. Pugliese A, Brown D, Garza D et al. Self-antigen-presenting cells expressing diabetes-associated autoantigens exist in both thymus and peripheral lymphoid organs. J Clin Invest 2001; 107(5):555-564.
233. Giannoukakis N, Bonham CA, Qian S et al. Prolongation of cardiac allograft survival using dendritic cells treated with NF-kB decoy oligodeoxyribonucleotides. Mol Ther 2000; 1(5 Pt 1):430-437.
234. Liu Y, Rabinovitch A, Suarez-Pinzon W et al. Expression of the bcl-2 gene from a defective HSV-1 amplicon vector protects pancreatic beta-cells from apoptosis. Hum Gene Ther 1996; 7(14):1719-1726.
235. Rabinovitch A, Suarez-Pinzon W, Strynadka K et al. Transfection of human pancreatic islets with an anti-apoptotic gene (bcl-2) protects beta-cells from cytokine-induced destruction. Diabetes 1999; 48(6):1223-1229.
236. Dupraz P, Rinsch C, Pralong WF et al. Lentivirus-mediated Bcl-2 expression in betaTC-tet cells improves resistance to hypoxia and cytokine-induced apoptosis while preserving in vitro and in vivo control of insulin secretion. Gene Ther 1999; 6(6):1160-1169.
237. Zhou YP, Pena JC, Roe MW et al. Overexpression of Bcl-x(L) in beta-cells prevents cell death but impairs mitochondrial signal for insulin secretion. Am J Physiol Endocrinol Metab 2000; 278(2):E340-351.
238. Ye J, Laychock SG. A protective role for heme oxygenase expression in pancreatic islets exposed to interleukin-1beta. Endocrinology 1998; 139(10):4155-4163.
239. Carpenter L, Cordery D, Biden TJ. Inhibition of protein kinase C delta protects rat INS-1 cells against interleukin-1beta and streptozotocin-induced apoptosis. Diabetes 2002; 51(2):317-324.
240. Dupraz P, Cottet S, Hamburger F et al. Dominant negative MyD88 proteins inhibit interleukin-1beta /interferon- gamma -mediated induction of nuclear factor kappa B-dependent nitrite production and apoptosis in beta cells. J Biol Chem 2000; 275(48):37672-37678.
241. Giannoukakis N, Mi Z, Rudert WA et al. Prevention of beta cell dysfunction and apoptosis activation in human islets by adenoviral gene transfer of the insulin-like growth factor I. Gene Ther 2000; 7(23):2015-2022.
242. Giannoukakis N, Rudert WA, Trucco M et al. Protection of human islets from the effects of interleukin-1beta by adenoviral gene transfer of an Ikappa B repressor. J Biol Chem 2000; 275(47):36509-36513.
243. Burkart V, Liu H, Bellmann K et al. Natural resistance of human beta cells toward nitric oxide is mediated by heat shock protein 70. J Biol Chem 2000; 275(26):19521-19528.
244. Grey ST, Arvelo MB, Hasenkamp W et al. A20 inhibits cytokine-induced apoptosis and nuclear factor kappaB- dependent gene activation in islets. J Exp Med 1999; 190(8):1135-1146.
245. Xu B, Moritz JT, Epstein PN. Overexpression of catalase provides partial protection to transgenic mouse beta cells. Free Radic Biol Med 1999; 27(7-8):830-837.
246. Benhamou PY, Moriscot C, Richard MJ et al. Adenovirus-mediated catalase gene transfer reduces oxidant stress in human, porcine and rat pancreatic islets. Diabetologia 1998; 41(9):1093-1100.
247. Hohmeier HE, Thigpen A, Tran VV et al. Stable expression of manganese superoxide dismutase (MnSOD) in insulinoma cells prevents IL-1beta- induced cytotoxicity and reduces nitric oxide production. J Clin Invest 1998; 101(9):1811-1820.
248. Rehman KK, Bertera S, Bottino R et al. Protection of islets by in situ peptide mediated transduction of the Ikappa B kinase (IKK) inhibitor nemo binding domain (NBD) peptide. J Biol Chem 2003; 9:9.
249. Gallichan WS, Kafri T, Krahl T et al. Lentivirus-mediated transduction of islet grafts with interleukin 4 results in sustained gene expression and protection from insulitis. Hum Gene Ther 1998; 9(18):2717-2726.
250. Smith DK, Korbutt GS, Suarez-Pinzon WL et al. Interleukin-4 or interleukin-10 expressed from adenovirus-transduced syngeneic islet grafts fails to prevent beta cell destruction in diabetic NOD mice. Transplantation 1997; 64(7):1040-1049.
251. Giannoukakis N, Rudert WA, Ghivizzani SC et al. Adenoviral gene transfer of the interleukin-1 receptor antagonist protein to human islets prevents IL-1beta-induced beta-cell impairment and activation of islet cell apoptosis in vitro. Diabetes 1999; 48(9):1730-1736.

252. Yasuda H, Nagata M, Arisawa K et al. Local expression of immunoregulatory IL-12p40 gene prolonged syngeneic islet graft survival in diabetic NOD mice. J Clin Invest 1998; 102(10):1807-1814.
253. Benhamou PY, Mullen Y, Shaked A et al. Decreased alloreactivity to human islets secreting recombinant viral interleukin 10. Transplantation 1996; 62(9):1306-1312.
254. Deng S, Ketchum RJ, Yang ZD et al. IL-10 and TGF-beta gene transfer to rodent islets: Effect on xenogeneic islet graft survival in naive and B-cell-deficient mice. Transplant Proc 1997; 29(4):2207-2208.
255. Hao W, Palmer JP. Recombinant human transforming growth factor beta does not inhibit the effects of interleukin-1 beta on pancreatic islet cells. J Interferon Cytokine Res 1995; 15(12):1075-1081.
256. Alexander AM, Crawford M, Bertera S et al. Indoleamine 2,3-dioxygenase expression in transplanted NOD Islets prolongs graft survival after adoptive transfer of diabetogenic splenocytes. Diabetes 2002; 51(2):356-365.
257. Gainer AL, Korbutt GS, Rajotte RV et al. Expression of CTLA4-Ig by biolistically transfected mouse islets promotes islet allograft survival. Transplantation 1997; 63(7):1017-1021.
258. Judge TA, Desai NM, Yang Z et al. Utility of adenoviral-mediated Fas ligand gene transfer to modulate islet allograft survival. Transplantation 1998; 66(4):426-434.
259. Kang SM, Schneider DB, Lin Z et al. Fas ligand expression in islets of Langerhans does not confer immune privilege and instead targets them for rapid destruction. Nat Med 1997; 3(7):738-743.
260. von Herrath MG, Efrat S, Oldstone MB et al. Expression of adenoviral E3 transgenes in beta cells prevents autoimmune diabetes. Proc Natl Acad Sci USA 1997; 94(18):9808-9813.
261. Mathieu C, Casteels K, Bouillon R et al. Protection against autoimmune diabetes in mixed bone marrow chimeras: Mechanisms involved. J Immunol 1997; 158(3):1453-1457.
262. Girman P, Kriz J, Dovolilova E et al. The effect of bone marrow transplantation on survival of allogeneic pancreatic islets with short-term tacrolimus conditioning in rats. Ann Transplant 2001; 6(2):43-45.
263. Seung E, Iwakoshi N, Woda BA et al. Allogeneic hematopoietic chimerism in mice treated with sublethal myeloablation and anti-CD154 antibody: Absence of graft-versus-host disease, induction of skin allograft tolerance, and prevention of recurrent autoimmunity in islet-allografted NOD/Lt mice. Blood 2000; 95(6):2175-2182.
264. Li H, Colson YL, Ildstad ST. Mixed allogeneic chimerism achieved by lethal and nonlethal conditioning approaches induces donor-specific tolerance to simultaneous islet allografts. Transplantation 1995; 60(6):523-529.
265. Li H, Ricordi C, Demetris AJ et al. Mixed xenogeneic chimerism (mouse+rat—>mouse) to induce donor-specific tolerance to sequential or simultaneous islet xenografts. Transplantation 1994; 57(4):592-598.
266. Rossini AA, Mordes JP, Greiner DL et al. Islet cell transplantation tolerance. Transplantation 2001; 72(8 Suppl):S43-46.
267. Ali A, Garrovillo M, Jin MX et al. Major histocompatibility complex class I peptide-pulsed host dendritic cells induce antigen-specific acquired thymic tolerance to islet cells. Transplantation 2000; 69(2):221-226.
268. Bertry-Coussot L, Lucas B, Danel C et al. Long-term reversal of established autoimmunity upon transient blockade of the LFA-1/intercellular adhesion molecule-1 pathway. J Immunol 2002; 168(7):3641-3648.
269. Georgiou HM, Brady JL, Silva A et al. Genetic modification of an islet tumor cell line inhibits its rejection. Transplant Proc 1997; 29(1-2):1032-1033.
270. Lew AM, Brady JL, Silva A et al. Secretion of CTLA4Ig by an SV40 T antigen-transformed islet cell line inhibits graft rejection against the neoantigen. Transplantation 1996; 62(1):83-89.
271. Weber CJ, Hagler MK, Chryssochoos JT et al. CTLA4-Ig prolongs survival of microencapsulated rabbit islet xenografts in spontaneously diabetic Nod mice. Transplant Proc 1996; 28(2):821-823.
272. Brady JL, Lew AM. Additive efficacy of CTLA4Ig and OX40Ig secreted by genetically modified grafts. Transplantation 2000; 69(5):724-730.
273. Sutherland RM, Brady JL, Georgiou HM et al. Protective effect of CTLA4Ig secreted by transgenic fetal pancreas allografts. Transplantation 2000; 69(9):1806-1812.

274. Goudy K, Song S, Wasserfall C et al. Adeno-associated virus vector-mediated IL-10 gene delivery prevents type 1 diabetes in NOD mice. Proc Natl Acad Sci USA 2001; 98(24):13913-13918.
275. Ko KS, Lee M, Koh JJ et al. Combined administration of plasmids encoding IL-4 and IL-10 prevents the development of autoimmune diabetes in nonobese diabetic mice. Mol Ther 2001; 4(4):313-316.
276. Koh JJ, Ko KS, Lee M et al. Degradable polymeric carrier for the delivery of IL-10 plasmid DNA to prevent autoimmune insulitis of NOD mice. Gene Ther 2000; 7(24):2099-2104.
277. Yang Z, Chen M, Wu R et al. Suppression of autoimmune diabetes by viral IL-10 gene transfer. J Immunol 2002; 168(12):6479-6485.
278. Zipris D, Karnieli E. A single treatment with IL-4 via retrovirally transduced lymphocytes partially protects against diabetes in BioBreeding (BB) rats. Jop 2002; 3(3):76-82.
279. Chang Y, Prud'homme GJ. Intramuscular administration of expression plasmids encoding interferon- gamma receptor/IgG1 or IL-4/IgG1 chimeric proteins protects from autoimmunity. J Gene Med 1999; 1(6):415-423.
280. Prud'homme GJ, Chang Y. Prevention of autoimmune diabetes by intramuscular gene therapy with a nonviral vector encoding an interferon-gamma receptor/IgG1 fusion protein. Gene Ther 1999; 6(5):771-777.
281. Piccirillo CA, Chang Y, Prud'homme GJ. TGF-beta1 somatic gene therapy prevents autoimmune disease in nonobese diabetic mice. J Immunol 1998; 161(8):3950-3956.
282. Balasa B, Boehm BO, Fortnagel A et al. Vaccination with glutamic acid decarboxylase plasmid DNA protects mice from spontaneous autoimmune diabetes and B7/CD28 costimulation circumvents that protection. Clin Immunol 2001; 99(2):241-252.
283. Jun HS, Chung YH, Han J et al. Prevention of autoimmune diabetes by immunogene therapy using recombinant vaccinia virus expressing glutamic acid decarboxylase. Diabetologia 2002; 45(5):668-676.
284. Efrat S, Serreze D, Svetlanov A et al. Adenovirus early region 3(E3) immunomodulatory genes decrease the incidence of autoimmune diabetes in NOD mice. Diabetes 2001; 50(5):980-984.
285. Weiner HL, Friedman A, Miller A et al. Oral tolerance: Immunologic mechanisms and treatment of animal and human organ-specific autoimmune diseases by oral administration of autoantigens. Annu Rev Immunol 1994; 12:809-837.
286. Polanski M, Melican NS, Zhang J et al. Oral administration of the immunodominant B-chain of insulin reduces diabetes in a cotransfer model of diabetes in the NOD mouse and is associated with a switch from Th1 to Th2 cytokines. J Autoimmun 1997; 10(4):339-346.
287. Bergerot I, Arreaza GA, Cameron MJ et al. Insulin B-chain reactive CD4+ regulatory T-cells induced by oral insulin treatment protect from type 1 diabetes by blocking the cytokine secretion and pancreatic infiltration of diabetogenic effector T-cells. Diabetes 1999; 48(9):1720-1729.
288. Prud'homme GJ, Chang Y, Li X. Immunoinhibitory DNA vaccine protects against autoimmune diabetes through cDNA encoding a selective CTLA-4 (CD152) ligand. Hum Gene Ther 2002; 13(3):395-406.
289. Gainer AL, Suarez-Pinzon WL, Min WP et al. Improved survival of biolistically transfected mouse islet allografts expressing CTLA4-Ig or soluble Fas ligand. Transplantation 1998; 66(2):194-199.
290. Welsh N, Oberg C, Hellerstrom C et al. Liposome mediated in vitro transfection of pancreatic islet cells. Biomed Biochim Acta 1990; 49(12):1157-1164.
291. Benhamou PY, Moriscot C, Prevost P et al. Standardization of procedure for efficient ex vivo gene transfer into porcine pancreatic islets with cationic liposomes. Transplantation 1997; 63(12):1798-1803.
292. Weber M, Deng S, Kucher T et al. Adenoviral transfection of isolated pancreatic islets: A study of programmed cell death (apoptosis) and islet function. J Surg Res 1997; 69(1):23-32.
293. Csete ME, Benhamou PY, Drazan KE et al. Efficient gene transfer to pancreatic islets mediated by adenoviral vectors. Transplantation 1995; 59(2):263-268.
294. Raper SE, DeMatteo RP. Adenovirus-mediated in vivo gene transfer and expression in normal rat pancreas. Pancreas 1996; 12(4):401-410.
295. Saldeen J, Curiel DT, Eizirik DL et al. Efficient gene transfer to dispersed human pancreatic islet cells in vitro using adenovirus-polylysine/DNA complexes or polycationic liposomes. Diabetes 1996; 45(9):1197-1203.

296. Giannoukakis N, Rudert WA, Ghivizzani SC et al. Adenoviral gene transfer of the interleukin-1 receptor antagonist protein to human islets prevents IL-1beta-induced beta-cell impairment and activation of islet cell apoptosis in vitro. Diabetes 1999; 48(9):1730-1736.
297. Muruve DA, Manfro RC, Strom TB et al. Ex vivo adenovirus-mediated gene delivery leads to long-term expression in pancreatic islet transplants. Transplantation 1997; 64(3):542-546.
298. Becker TC, BeltrandelRio H, Noel RJ et al. Overexpression of hexokinase I in isolated islets of Langerhans via recombinant adenovirus. Enhancement of glucose metabolism and insulin secretion at basal but not stimulatory glucose levels. J Biol Chem 1994; 269(33):21234-21238.
299. Giannoukakis N, Rudert WA, Trucco M et al. Protection of human islets from the effects of interleukin-1beta by adenoviral gene transfer of an IkappaB repressor. J Biol Chem 2000.
300. Kapturczak M, Zolotukhin S, Cross J et al. Transduction of human and mouse pancreatic islet cells using a bicistronic recombinant adeno-associated viral vector. Mol Ther 2002; 5(2):154-160.
301. Shifrin AL, Auricchio A, Yu QC et al. Adenoviral vector-mediated insulin gene transfer in the mouse pancreas corrects streptozotocin-induced hyperglycemia. Gene Ther 2001; 8(19):1480-1489.
302. Uchikoshi F, Yang ZD, Rostami S et al. Prevention of autoimmune recurrence and rejection by adenovirus- mediated CTLA4Ig gene transfer to the pancreatic graft in BB rat. Diabetes 1999; 48(3):652-657.
303. Moriscot C, Pattou F, Kerr-Conte J et al. Contribution of adenoviral-mediated superoxide dismutase gene transfer to the reduction in nitric oxide-induced cytotoxicity on human islets and INS-1 insulin-secreting cells. Diabetologia 2000; 43(5):625-631.
304. Guo Z, Shen J, Mital D et al. Efficient gene transfer and expression in islets by an adenoviral vector that lacks all viral genes. Cell Transplant 1999; 8(6):661-671.
305. Leibowitz G, Beattie GM, Kafri T et al. Gene transfer to human pancreatic endocrine cells using viral vectors. Diabetes 1999; 48(4):745-753.
306. Ju Q, Edelstein D, Brendel MD et al. Transduction of nondividing adult human pancreatic beta cells by an integrating lentiviral vector. Diabetologia 1998; 41(6):736-739.
307. Giannoukakis N, Mi Z, Gambotto A et al. Infection of intact human islets by a lentiviral vector. Gene Ther 1999; 6(9):1545-1551.
308. Mi Z, Mai J, Lu X, Robbins PD. Characterization of a class of cationic peptides able to facilitate efficient protein transduction in vitro and in vivo. Mol Ther 2000; 2(4):339-347.

Chapter 3

Immunogene Therapy with Nonviral Vectors

Ciriaco A. Piccirillo, Argyrios N. Theofilopoulos and Gérald J. Prud'homme*

Introduction

The majority of gene therapy studies have been performed with viral vectors that present important limitations in terms of immunogenicity and pathogenicity. Nonviral (usually plasmid-based) gene therapy is not hampered by these limitations and, although gene transfer is generally less efficient, it has been successfully employed in the prevention or treatment of several experimental autoimmune diseases.[1-12] Gene transfer of naked DNA can be enhanced by several methods and, at least for some applications, can now rival or even surpass viral gene transfer. Indeed, in animal models of disease, nonviral methods are effective at delivering cDNA encoding regulatory cytokines such as IL-10 or transforming growth factor β1 (TGF-β1), which exert many anti-inflammatory effects and promote the activity of regulatory T cells (Tr). This approach is also effective for the administration of cytokine inhibitors such as IL-1 receptor antagonist (IL-1Ra), soluble interferon gamma (IFNγ) receptor (IFNγR)/IgG-Fc fusion protein, or TNFα receptor (TNFR).[9-12] Furthermore, in vivo transfer of nucleic acid segments (or plasmid-based delivery of these molecules), such as cytosine-phosphate-guanine (CpG)-containing oligodeoxynucleotides (ODNs) or small inhibitory RNA (siRNA), is highly promising in the therapy of conditions as diverse as autoimmune diseases, other inflammatory disorders, allergy, infectious diseases and cancer. In this chapter, we will focus primarily on nonviral gene therapy of autoimmune diseases and other inflammatory disorders, although applications to other diseases will be mentioned when relevant.

The design of effective immunotherapies must include determination of the immune mechanisms directly responsible for inflammatory tissue injury. In this respect, significant pathology can be attributed to the inflammatory cytokines IL-1, TNFα, IL-12 and IFNγ, or molecularly related cytokines.[13-20] Moreover, any combination of these cytokines is likely to be even more injurious than each component alone. IL-1, TNFα and IL-12 are produced principally by macrophages and dendritic cells, whereas IFNγ is produced by T-helper (Th) type 1 (Th1) cells, cytotoxic T lymphocytes (CTLs) and natural killer (NK) cells. For example, in nonobese diabetic (NOD) mice with autoimmune diabetes (type 1 diabetes [T1D]), mononuclear infiltration of the islets of Langerhans (insulitis) is associated with local IL-12 and IFNγ production reflecting, at least in part, a Th1-dependent reaction.[19,20] Similarly, Th1-mediated inflammatory pathology has been observed in experimental autoimmune encephalomyelitis (EAE), and this disease can be passively transferred with autoagressive Th1

*Gérald J. Prud'homme—Department of Laboratory Medicine and Pathobiology, University of Toronto and St. Michael's Hospital, 30 Bond Street, Room 2013CC, Toronto, Canada M5B1W8. Email: prudhommeg@smh.toronto.on.ca

Gene Therapy of Autoimmune Disease, edited by Gérald J. Prud'homme. ©2005 Eurekah.com and Kluwer Academic / Plenum Publishers.

clones reacting to either myelin basic protein (MBP), proteolipid protein (PLP), or other central nervous system (CNS) antigens.[21,22]

Clinically, the neutralization of TNFα with monoclonal antibodies (mAbs) or soluble receptors has proven effective in the treatment of rheumatoid arthritis (RA),[14-17] and this represents one of the most effective immunotherapies designed in recent years. Consequently, gene therapists have attempted to ameliorate autoimmune diseases by neutralizing the activity of inflammatory cytokines. Obviously, as shown in RA, this can also be accomplished with protein drugs such as mAbs or recombinant receptors. However, these proteins have to be repeatedly administered in large amounts by parenteral routes. MAbs are also subject to neutralization by the recipient's immune response, even though this can be reduced by "humanization" of the antibodies. As an alternative to direct anticytokine therapy, it is feasible to administer regulatory cytokines (e.g., IL-4, IL-10 or TGF-β) which inhibit the production of inflammatory mediators. Unfortunately, the use of cytokines as protein therapeutic agents is also markedly problematic because they are expensive to produce, have short half-lives, and frequently exert toxic effects, especially when administered as a bolus.

Gene therapy offers the possibility of eliminating or diminishing some of these problems. It permits long-term, relatively constant delivery of anti-inflammatory or immunoregulatory mediators. In the case of cytokines, this can be accomplished at low levels which are less likely to be toxic. Specific tissues can be targeted, such as the joints or the CNS. Very recent studies suggest that the production of pathogenic inflammatory mediators can be inhibited with gene-specific short (small) inhibitory RNAs (siRNAs). Furthermore, as discussed in other chapters, appropriate genes can be transduced into autoantigen-specific T cells ex vivo. These cells can then be injected into diseased animals, where they specifically infiltrate the antigen-bearing target organ, and downregulate autoimmune processes.

Nonviral Gene Therapy Vectors

Almost all the nonviral vectors employed thus far are expression plasmids, which have been designed for high expression in striated muscle cells or other cells. The construction of these vectors is quite simple and straightforward. The best plasmids carry a strong promoter (most of often the human cytomegalovirus (CMV) immediate-early enhancer promoter [IE-EP]), an intron (such as CMV intron A), a multiple cloning site for insertion of the gene of interest, and an appropriate transcriptional terminator segment.

The construction and in vivo delivery of these vectors has been extensively reviewed,[8-11] and will only be briefly described here. The transfer of naked plasmid DNA following needle injection occurs more readily in skeletal muscle than in most other tissues.[10,11] Furthermore, in various tissues, transfection has been enhanced or accomplished by "gene gun" delivery (usually DNA-coated gold particles propelled into cells),[23] jet injection of DNA,[24,25] cationic polymers such as polyethylenimine (PEI) and poly-L-lysine (PLL), and cationic liposomes.[25] Recently, in vivo electroporation has been shown to be one of the most effective approaches.[25-28] In addition, infusion of plasmids under pressure in veins or arteries (hydrodynamic delivery) results in the extensive transfection of cells in tissues supplied by the relevant vasculature, such as liver or muscle.[27,29,30] Indeed, hydrodynamic approaches are advantageous when the transfection of very large number of cells in a tissue is desired. Although some hydrodynamic approaches are not feasible in humans, due to the large amount of fluid that is rapidly infused, modified approaches (especially on isolated limbs) appear clinically applicable.[31] Interestingly, ultrasound has also been employed to enhance gene delivery,[32-34] but has been less effective than either electroporation or hydrodynamic delivery. Nevertheless, various physical methods can be combined (electroporation and ultrasound or other combinations), to further improve transfection.[34]

Optimizing Gene Transfer

Skeletal muscle represents an advantageous target for nonviral gene therapy, as first demonstrated by Wolff and his colleagues.[35,36] It accounts for 30-50% of the body weight, and is easily accessible and abundantly vascularized. Moreover, transgene expression is generally much more prolonged than in other tissues, probably because striated myocytes are nondividing, long-lived cells. In mice, we observed that protein production reaches a maximum after the injection of 50-100 μg of naked plasmid DNA per muscle.[11] Without any special maneuvers to enhance transfection, 50 μg of DNA can lead to the synthesis of > 300 ng of nonsecreted reporter protein (e.g., luciferase).[37] In the case of secreted proteins, serum values can range from a few picograms/ml to > 300 ng/ml.[2-5,38] Not surprisingly, several factors affect these results, including vector components (e.g., promoters, introns and terminator sequences) and the rate of protein turnover. Maximum protein levels are most frequently recorded 1 to 2 weeks after DNA administration, but the persistence of expression varies greatly depending on the antigenicity of the product and other factors. The presence of unmethylated CpG motifs (see below) in the vector has an inflammatory effect which contributes to the shut down of expression, and the inclusion of genes encoding inflammatory cytokines is likely to have a similar negative effect.

In mice, the injection of a 50 μl dose of fluorescence-labeled plasmid into the tibialis anterior muscle is followed by the rapid diffusion of DNA throughout the muscle.[39] DNA is internalized by myocytes within 5 min, and over several hours by mononuclear cells (perhaps macrophages or dendritic cells) located along muscle fibers and in the draining lymph nodes. Notably, the transgene is expressed primarily by muscle cells,[39] but DNA vaccination studies suggest that dendritic cells (DCs) are also transfected, particularly when electroporation is applied. Since DCs are present in small numbers in normal muscle, this is not easy to demonstrate. The mechanism by which plasmids travel from the extracellular space to the nuclei of skeletal muscle cells remains unclear. However, it may be of relevance that these cells are multinucleated and the nuclei are located peripherally, in apposition to the cell membrane.

In Vivo Electroporation

Numerous studies[5,25-28,39-54] have shown that in vivo low voltage electroporation greatly augments transfection. Thus, electrogene transfer (EGT) increased reporter protein production in muscle by 100-fold or more in some studies. Electric pulses are thought to increase DNA entry into cells by creating transient pores in the cell membrane, and by promoting DNA motility (electrophoretic effect). Electroporation is a versatile approach, and has been successfully used to enhance DNA transfer into muscle (heart, skeletal),[26,39-47,54] liver,[50] brain,[51] various tumors, testis, bladder, embryos and other tissues.[31,34,35,53] This technique is an adaptation of electrochemotherapy (ECT), where in vivo electroporation (electropermeabilization) promotes entry of some anti-cancer drugs (e.g., Bleomycin) into cells, presumably due to the formation of transient pores in cell membranes.[54-58] ECT has been effective in animal models and clinical trials. Furthermore, ECT and EGT have been successfully combined for anti-tumor therapy.[58]

To enhance intramuscular gene transfer, electrical pulses using invasive or noninvasive electrodes are applied at the site of, and shortly after, DNA injection.[5,34,54] Optimally, this consists of low field strength (100-200 V/cm), relatively long (20-50 milliseconds) squarewave electric pulses, applied 6-8 times in quick succession. These values are based on our own experience, but are similar to those reported by most other authors. These low-voltage electrical pulses cause muscle damage, but it is usually mild and transient. For instance, Mathiesen[43] examined muscles 3 days after injection of DNA and electroporation under various conditions, and observed regions of necrotic fibers of increasing extent with increasing cumulative pulse duration. The majority of surviving fibers expressed the reporter gene. Two weeks after electroporation the muscles appeared grossly normal. He noted the presence of muscle fibers with central nuclei, most likely indicating muscle regeneration from satellite cells.

CpG Motifs and Toll-Like Receptor 9 (Tlr9)

An important component of the plasmid is the presence of unmethylated CpG-containing immunostimulatory sequences (ISS), that can activate innate immunity by binding to TLR9 located in endocytic vesicles of APCs.[59-61] Engagement of TLR9 triggers a cell signaling cascade involving sequentially myeloid differentiation primary response gene 88 (MyD88), interleukin-1 receptor activated kinase (IRAK), tumour necrosis factor receptor (TNFR)-associated factor 6 (TRAF6), and activation of NFκB.[59] Cells that express TLR9, which include plasmacytoid dendritic cells (PDCs) and B cells, produce interferon α and β (IFNaβ), inflammatory cytokines such as IL-12, and chemokines.

PDCs represent a small subpopulation of cells with the ability to produce large amounts of IFNαβ,[62,63] which promotes a Th1 response. It appears that the early (innate) production of IFNαβ at the beginning of an immune response stimulates $CD8^+$ T-cell proliferation and promotes activation of NK cells. CpG-stimulated DCs produce IL-12 which activates acquired antigen-specific T cell responses. There are important inter-species differences, in that in humans only PDCs and B cells express TLR9 (although other cells respond to TLR9 engagement, presumably by indirect stimulation), while in mice cells of other phenotypes, such as monocytes, macrophages and myeloid DCs, also express this receptor.[62-63] These differences are likely to influence the outcome of DNA vaccination and are highly relevant to vaccine design.

Optimal CpG motifs for activating mouse or rabbit immune cells have the general formula, purine-purine-CG-pyrimidine-pyrimidine.[59-61] However, for activating human cells, and cells of several other species, the optimal motif is TCGTT and/or TCGTA. In addition, some sequences that are immediately adjacent to these short motifs can contribute to the immunostimulatory effects.[59] Three classes of CpG-containing oligodeoxynucleotides (ODNs) have been described.[59-61] CpG ODNs of the B-class (also called K-class) strongly stimulate B cells, promote PDC maturation, but induce only low amounts of IFNαβ. In contrast, A-class (also called D-class) ODNs strongly stimulate plasmacytoid DCs (PDCs) to secrete IFNαβ, but are poor at activating B cells. C-Class ODNs combine the properties of the A and B classes, and are very strong Th1 adjuvants. The high levels of IFNα induced by either A-class or C-class ODNs activate NK cells efficiently. Moreover, CpG ODNs promote the transition from monocytes to myeloid DCs, and contribute to DC maturation.

Not all CpG ODNs are stimulatory. Suppressive motifs have also been described and they are rich in polyG or -GC sequences, tend to be methylated, and are present in the DNA of mammals and certain viruses.[60] These neutralizing motifs (CpG-N motifs) also exit in plasmids. Most DNA vaccines contain numerous CpG motifs, some of which are in an immunostimulatory context, while others are inhibitory. Thus, the ultimate effect of the plasmid DNA backbone in DNA vaccination may depend on the ratio of stimulatory and inhibitory sequences. Indeed, Klinman and his colleagues[64,65] report that the immunostimulatory activity of CpG ODNs can be abrogated in vitro and in vivo by the addition of suppressive sequences. It appears that stimulatory and suppressive ODNs bind to the same cells, and suppression tends to be dominant. When both types of sequences are joined recognition proceeds in a 5' to 3' direction, such that a 5' motif can interfere with one that is located immediately downstream. Suppressive motifs interfere with the maturation of endosomal vesicles and the colocalization of CpG ODNs and TLR9 in these vesicles. Interestingly, suppressive ODNs can protect against CpG-induced lesions, such as arthritis.[65]

The innate immune response created by CpG ISS is desirable for DNA vaccination, since it promotes the maturation of DCs and primes T cells to respond to the relevant antigen. However, CpG motifs are detrimental in gene therapy studies. First, their nonspecific inflammatory effects might directly injure tissues,and/or confuse the interpretation of immunological studies.Second, the CMV IE-EP, and other viral promoters, are turned off by inflammatory cytokines (particularly IFNγ and TNFα).[66-68] Since most plasmids carry large numbers of

CpG motifs, it is not easy to eliminate them completely. Nevertherless, some recently available commercial plasmid vectors are devoid of CpG elements, even in sequences coding for reporter genes (e.g., InVivogen, San Diego, CA). This is possible because of the eight codons that contain CG, all can be substituted by at least two other codons that code for the same amino acid. Moreover, it appears that CpG motifs bind to TLR9 only in an unmethylated form. A recent study[69] revealed that methylation of plasmids abrogates CpG/TLR9 interactions, while retaining vector expression. Mice inoculated with a CpG-methylated plasmid expressing a viral protein showed delayed clearance of transfected cells and failed to mount a strong immune response to the viral product. Importantly, the persistence of vector expression was increased.

An alternative approach involves deletion of most vector elements, to produce minicircles containing only, or primarily, the expression cassette.[70,71] These small vectors transfect cells more efficiently, presumably because of their small size. Furthermore, they lack all the CpG sequences of the vector backbone, and retain only those that might be present in essential transcriptional elements (these can also be replaced with alternative codons). Minicircle DNA vectors are remarkable for the level and persistence of transgene expression. Indeed, minicircular DNAs lacking bacterial sequences expressed 45- and 560-fold more serum human factor IX and alpha1-antitrypsin, respectively, compared to standard plasmid DNAs transfected into mouse liver.[70] Undoubtedly, vectors that have been modified for a reduction in CpG motifs will have significant advantages for many forms of gene therapy, where the activation of innate immunity is not desirable. On the other hand, CpG motifs may be beneficial in the treatment of allergic diseases (see below), or in cancer gene therapy.

CpG ODNs as Immunotherapeutic Agents

CpG ODNs are finding increasing applications for immunotherapy (Table 1). The ability of ODNs carrying immununostimulatory CpG motifs (or ISS) to activate innate immune mechanisms has proven valuable in cancer immunotherapy.[59,60] Importantly, the ODNs stimulate DCs and induce their maturation. These DCs are more effective at stimulating effector T cells and, furthermore, they secrete cytokines such as IL-6 which appear to protect effector cells against the suppressive effects of regulatory T cells.[72] ISS can also stimulate NK cells and B cells, which contributes to anti-tumor immunity in some models.

Table 1. Examples of therapeutic applications of nucleic acid therapy with CpG or siRNA

Therapeutic Agent	Disease Model	References
CpG ODNs	DC maturation/cancer immunotherapy	59, 60, 80-82
	Blocking the effects of regulatory T cells	72
	Experimental asthma	76-82
	Allergic conjunctivitis	75
siRNA	Gene silencing in the liver	191, 192
(synthetic or	Protection against induced hepatic necrosis	193, 194
vector-based)	Protection against viral hepatitis	199
	Anti-HIV-1 therapy	198
	Gene silencing in limb muscles	195, 196
	Cancer immunotherapy	184-187

CpG, cytosine-phosphate-guanine; DC, dendritic cells; HIV-1, human immunodeficiency virus type 1; ODNs, oligodeoxynucleotides; siRNA, short (small) interfering RNA.

CpGs have also been applied to the therapy of allergic diseases.[73-81] The CpG-ODN can be coadministered with the allergen, or directly fused with that molecule. Notably, ovalbumin (OVA) conjugated to a CpG-ODN and administered intratracheally in mice was found to be 100-fold more effective at ameliorating OVA-induced asthma than a mixture of OVA and CpG-ODN.[79,80] It is unclear why conjugation is more effective, but this may be related to increased uptake of the antigen by APCs, or colocalization of both molecules to the same APC. ODNs can alter Th1/Th2 balance in a favorable way (decreased Th2), possibly by stimulating production of Th1-type inflammatory cytokines such as IL-12 and IFNγ.[79-81] In allergic diseases, at least three major modalities have produced positive therapeutic effects: (1) DNA vaccination against allergens; (2) immunization with allergen/ODN mixtures or allergen/ODN conjugates; and (3) administration of ODNs alone.

Several authors have documented that CpG-ODN therapy inhibits Th2 cytokine production, eosinophilic inflammation and airway hypersensitivity in murine models of asthma.[76-81] The inhibition of eosinophilia is thought to be related to decreased IL-5 production (a Th2 cytokine). CpG ODNs were also found to be remarkably effective against allergic conjunctivitis.[75] Although most literature has focused on Th1/Th2 antagonism, the role of Th1 cells can be questioned, because CpG ODNs were protective against airway hypersensitivity in mice lacking IL-12 and IFNγ[82] Indeed, some ODNs have been reported to induce IL-10, and protection against allergy might depend on the activity of IL-10-producing regulatory T cells, or other types of regulatory cells.[82] In a murine model of chronic asthma, CpG ODNs also increased the amount of TGF-β1 in bronchoalveolar lavage fluid, possibly due to the action of Tr cells.[78] However, it remains unclear which features of ODNs would make them suitable for the induction of regulatory cytokines, rather than inflammatory cytokines.

Detrimental Effects of Plasmid DNA or CpG ISS Motifs

It is of some concern that transfected muscle cells may be attacked and injured by the immune system following DNA vaccination against foreign antigens, and indeed this has been reported.[83] A related concern is the production of pathogenic anti-DNA antibodies, potentially induced by plasmid DNA and its ISS motifs, but the risk appears relatively small. Indeed, B cells have mechanisms which prevent autoantibody production in response to CpG stimulation,[84] although this tolerance can be broken.[85] In lupus-prone mice, anti-dsDNA antibodies titers are increased by DNA vaccination. Surprisingly, lupus-like disease was either not altered or reduced in some studies.[86,87] However, recent reports indicate that stimulation through TLR9 induces progression of renal disease in MRL-*lpr/lpr* (Fas deficient)[88] and NZB x NZWF1[89] lupus-prone mice. Evidently, special caution should be exercised in administering CpG-bearing plasmids to patients with autoimmune diseases.

Local injection of stimulatory ODNs can induce inflammation. For instance intra-articular injection of these ODNs induces a form of arthritis, characterized by joint swelling, synovial hyperplasia and leukocytic infiltration.[90,91] Interestingly, this form of arthritis is reduced by prior systemic administration of suppressive ODNs.[90,91]

The Potent Inhibitory Effects of TGF-β1 and Its Use in Gene Therapy

The most potent anti-inflammatory cytokine is TGF-β1, though IL-4, IL-10, and IL-13 have some similar effects, particularly through their action on macrophages. There is a plethora of information in the literature on the immunobiology of TGF-β,[6,92-102] and only major points are mentioned here. At least three TGF-β isoforms exist in mammals, but TGF-β1 is the principal type produced by cells of the immune system. It is secreted in a latent form where mature TGF-β1 is associated with a precursor peptide (latency associated peptide (LAP) and latent TGF-β1-binding protein (LTBP). The active form can be generated in vitro by acidification of this complex, and is probably released in vivo through the action of plasmin and other proteases in inflammatory or other sites, though the mechanism is not fully elucidated. TGF-β1 receptors are expressed by almost all cells and, interestingly, this cytokine also binds to several matrix components in tissue. It has fibrogenic and angiogenic effects that contribute to wound healing.[92,102]

TGF-β1 is produced by regulatory T cells (Tr), particularly those designated Th3 and Tr1 (reviewed in refs. 95-98, 103). Importantly, TGF-β has also emerged as an important differentiation factor for Tr cells.[95-98,104-109] In addition, this cytokine is produced by macrophages and many other cell types in various tissues. It exerts diverse immunoinhibitory effects on B lymphocytes, $CD4^+$ T lymphocytes (Th1 or Th2), CTLs, NK cells, lymphokine-activated killer (LAK) cells, and macrophages.[6,95-97] In macrophages, TGF-β1 antagonizes the activities of IFNγ and TNFα, and inhibits inducible nitric oxide synthase (iNOS) activity. This cytokine also alters expression of E-selectin and other adhesion molecules, and interferes with the adhesion of neutrophils and lymphocytes to endothelial cells. The potent immunosuppressive effects of TGF-β1 are most clearly demonstrated in studies of knockout (KO) mice, which die rapidly from a multi-organ inflammatory syndrome.

The fibrogenic and immunosuppressive effects of TGF-β1 overproduction have been linked to several pathologic conditions, particularly pulmonary fibrosis, glomerulopathy, systemic sclerosis, and chronic graft-versus-host disease (GVHD).[6,102,110] This cytokine promotes corneal opacification (increased extracellular matrix, angiogenesis, cell infiltration) after injury or transplantation. Moreover, it is produced by most tumours, where it is capable of blocking anti-tumor immunity.[111] High production of TGF-β1 has also been noted in chronic infectious diseases, where it hampers the elimination of pathogens.[112] On the other hand, injection of a plasmid encoding TGF-β1 into skin wounds improved healing in diabetic mice.[113] This might be related to the stimulation of fibroblast proliferation and collagen deposition, as well as the promotion of angiogenesis.

Cytokine Gene Therapy of Lupus

Administration of TGF-β1 is protective in several inflammatory conditions. In rodents, microgram amounts of either active or latent protein are required to achieve immunosuppressive effects.[114-116] The delivery of TGF-β1 by gene transfer has been examined by several authors in classical models of autoimmunity or inflammatory disease (Table 2). We have shown that, among other advantages, this route obviates the time consuming and expensive process of

Table 2. Examples of successful plasmid-based TGF-β1 gene therapy

Disease	Method/Vector	References
Autoimmune diabetes	Naked pDNA (i.m.)	1
EAE	Naked pDNA (i.m.)	3
EAE	CNS-localized DNA-liposome	138
Murine lupus	Naked pDNA (i.m.)	117, 118
Induced colitis	pDNA (i.m. or intranasal)	126, 127
SCW-induced arthritis	Naked pDNA (i.m.)	128
Cardiac allograft rejection	Direct intracardiac injection (naked DNA), or perfusion of heart with DNA-liposome complex	129-132
Wound healing	Application of naked DNA to wound	113

CNS, central nervous system; EAE, experimental autoimmune encephalomyelitis; i.m. pDNA, intra-muscular injection of naked plasmid DNA: TGF-β1, transforming growth factor β1; SCW, streptococcal cell wall.

TGF-β1 purification. Intramuscular (i.m.) injection of naked plasmid DNA encoding latent TGF-β1 (pCMV-TGF-β1) increases circulating levels of this cytokine by several folds, suppresses delayed-type hypersensitivity (DTH) and protects against autoimmune lesions.[1,3,117,118] In most cases, a gene encoding latent TGF-β1 has been employed, and it is evident that the cytokine is released into the circulation and activated in vivo, although the mechanism of activation has not been clearly established. We hypothesize that at least part of the circulating TGF-β1 is activated at sites of inflammation, through the action of macrophages or other lymphoid cells. Although administration of a modified active form of the TGF-β1 gene is feasible, the fact that virtually all cells have receptors[102] makes it likely that most of the TGF-β1 molecules would never reach their intended target, and numerous adverse effects would likely occur.

Raz and colleagues[117,118] showed that direct injections of cDNA expression plasmids encoding IL-2, IL-4, or latent TGF-β1 into mouse skeletal muscle induce biological effects characteristic of these cytokines. Mice injected intramuscularly with a vector encoding IL-2 had enhanced humoral and cellular immune responses to an exogenous antigen, transferrin, which was delivered at a separate site. These IL-2 effects were abolished by coadministration of a vector directing synthesis of TGF-β1. The TGF-β1 vector alone depressed the anti-transferrin antibody response and caused an 8-fold increase in plasma TGF-β1 activity. The TGF-β1 plasmid injection did not cause muscle infiltration with monocytes or neutrophils and there was no evidence for fibrotic changes. Monthly injections of TGF-β1 plasmid DNA in these mice between 6 and 26 weeks of age prolonged survival of 70% at 26 weeks compared with 40% in the control group, decreased anti-chromatin and rheumatoid factor antibodies and induced a 50% decrease in total IgG production. Renal function was improved with reduced BUN levels and kidney inflammation as estimated by a histology, and these beneficial effects occurred in the apparent absence of local or systemic side effects. In contrast, injection of IL-2 cDNA resulted in decreased survival to 20% at 26 weeks, enhanced total IgG synthesis and autoantibody production with a 4.5-fold increase in anti-chromatin antibodies.

However, not all investigators have found IL-2 to be detrimental in lupus. For example, Gutierrez-Ramos and colleagues[119] observed a beneficial effect for IL-2 on the disease progression in MRL *lpr/lpr* mice using live vaccinia recombinant viruses expressing the human IL-2 gene, e.g., prolonged survival, decreased autoantibody and rheumatoid factor titres, marked attenuation of kidney interstitial infiltration and intraglomerular proliferation, as well as clearance of synovial mononuclear infiltrates. Additionally, such inoculation resulted in drastically reduced double-negative T cells, improved thymic differentiation and restored normal values of mature cells in peripheral lymphoid organs. A caveat is that immune responses to vaccinia antigens could have altered the immune system and contributed to this beneficial effect. Indeed, the use of strongly antigenic viral vectors is a serious limitation for immunological studies.

Huggins and colleagues[120,121] also studied the effects of IL-2 and TGF-β gene therapy on the progress of autoimmune disease in MRL *lpr/lpr* mice, using a different approach. The mice were treated orally with a nonpathogenic strain of *Salmonella typhimurium* bearing the aroA-aroD- mutations and carrying the murine genes encoding IL-2 or TGF-β1. This results in the in vivo uptake of the bacteria by some cells (e.g., phagocytes), gene transfer, synthesis and slow release of the cytokines, although the intracellular mechanisms of gene transfer are not fully elucidated. These investigators reported that, contrary to expectation, TGF-β1 gene therapy failed to ameliorate disease and generally produced effects opposite to those of IL-2 therapy. IL-2 restored the deficient T-cell proliferative response to mitogen and suppressed the autoantibody response and glomerulonephritis.

These conflicting results demonstrate the risks involved in using cytokines as therapeutic molecules. Most cytokines have complex pleiotropic actions, and may have stimulatory or inhibitory effects depending on their concentration, target tissue or cell, as well as interacting cytokines in the extra-cellular milieu. Indeed, the coactivity of multiple cytokines produced in inflammatory sites may produce effects that have never been documented in vitro. As a result, cytokines that are generally thought of as anti-inflammatory, such as TGF-β1, sometimes have inflammatory effects.[6,122] Similarly, inflammatory cytokines, such as IL-12, are sometimes paradoxically protective. For example Hagiwara and colleagues[123] found that administering a DNA plasmid encoding IL-12 to MRL-*lpr/lpr* mice significantly inhibited lymphadenopathy and splenomegaly. A significant decrease in serum IgG anti-DNA autoantibody titres was observed, and plasmid IL-12 therapy was also associated with a reduction in the proteinuria and glomerulonephritis. Serum IFNγ level was increased by inoculating the IL-12 encoding plasmid, suggesting that the cytokine balance was skewed towards a Th1-type response. This is surprising, since other authors found that neutralizing IFNγ is protective in this disease (see below). It may be that this plasmid also induced the production of regulatory cytokines that counterbalanced inflammatory cytokines, but we can only speculate on the mechanism at this point.

Recent studies also show that IFNγ can induce the expression of PD-1 ligand 1 (PD-L1) on DCs, endothelial cells, and other cells.[124] This ligand binds to the inhibitory molecule PD-1 and turns off T-cell and B-cell responses. Other inhibitory receptors such as B and T lymphocyte attenuator (BTLA) show many similarities.[125] Therefore, inflammatory cytokines may paradoxically activate negative regulatory mechanisms which protect against autoimmunity.

Applicability of TGF-β1 Gene Therapy to Various Inflammatory Diseases

In addition to lupus, administration of TGF-β1 is protective in several inflammatory conditions (Table 2). Kitani et al[126] showed that a single intranasal dose of a plasmid encoding active TGF-β1 in mice prevented the development of Th1-dependent colitis induced by the haptenating reagent, 2,4, 6-trinitrobenzene sulfonic acid (TNBS). Plasmid administration abrogated TNBS colitis after it had been established, and it led to the expression of TGF-β1 mRNA in the intestinal lamina propria, as well as the appearance of TGF-β1-producing T cells and macrophages in these tissues. These cells caused marked suppression of IL-12 and IFNγ production and enhancement of IL-10 production. Thus, TGF-β1 gene therapy appears to augment the production of TGF-β1 by various cells, including regulatory T cells. Interestingly, this therapy was not associated with fibrosis.

In a similar model of induced rat colitis, i.m. injection of a TGF-β1 expression plasmid also ameliorated colonic inflammation and ulceration.[127] On histological examination, 50% of TGF-β1-plasmid treated rats had minimal or no ulceration and a significant decrease in mucosal leukotriene C4 generation, whereas 83% of control plasmid-treated rats had a maximal damage score. Similarly, others[128] administered a TGF-β1 plasmid to rats with streptococcal cell wall (SCW)-induced arthritis. Systemic delivery of TFG-β1 initiated by i.m. injection of a single dose of 300 μg of plasmid DNA encoding TGF-β1, but not vector DNA, profoundly suppressed the subsequent evolution of chronic erosive disease. However, it should be noted that, unlike systemic administration, the intra-articular delivery of TGF-β1 can induce osteoarthritis-like inflammation.[122] This may be related to the chemotactic, angiogenic and fibrogenic properties of this cytokine.

TGF-β1 gene therapy might also be applicable to the prevention of transplant rejection. Indeed, direct injection of plasmids encoding this cytokine into cardiac muscle protected mice against allogeneic heart transplant rejection.[129-131] Plasmid-induced immunosuppression was localized to the area of the graft because plasmid injected remote from the graft was not protective, and systemic immunity was not affected. Similarly, the perfusion of donor hearts with DNA-liposome carrying the TGF-β1 gene prolonged allograft survival in approximately two-thirds of recipients.[132] This was associated with reduced Th1 responses and an inhibition of alloantibody isotype switching. Transgene expression persisted for at least 60 days; however, long-term transfected allografts exhibited exacerbated fibrosis and neointimal development.

Table 3. Examples of plasmid-based IL-4 or IL-10 gene therapy

Cytokine	Disease	References
IL-4, or	Autoimmune diabetes	4, 136
IL-4/IgG-Fc	EAE	3, 138
	CIA	176
IL-10, or	Autoimmune diabetes	147, 148
vIL-10/IgG-Fc	Myocarditis	152-154
	Thyroiditis (EAT)	155, 156
	CIA	177, 178
Combined IL-4 and IL-10	Autoimmune diabetes	149, 150

CIA, collagen-induced arthritis; EAE, experimental autoimmune encephalomyelitis; EAT, experimental autoimmune thyroiditis.

Cytokine Gene Therapy of Organ-Specific Autoimmune Diseases

We found that the injection of a TGF-β1 plasmid (100 μg/muscle in 2-4 muscles every 2 weeks; into the tibialis anterior or rectus femoris) considerably reduced the incidence of diabetes in NOD mice.[1] In the cyclophosphamide (CYP)-accelerated form of this disease, there was a four-fold reduction in incidence. In nonCYP-treated mice (natural course), treatment reduced the incidence of diabetes by approximately 50 % over the course of several weeks, even when therapy was administered late in mice that already had insulitis. Semi-quantitative analysis of cytokine mRNA expression in the pancreas of treated mice revealed decreased levels of inflammatory cytokine mRNA. Detrimental effects were not noted and, in this respect, the use of latent TGF-β1 is probably an advantage since it can only act in sites where it can be activated, such as inflammatory lesions.

IL-4 and IL-10 have also been extensively studied as possible immunotherapeutic cytokines. Systemic administration of IL-4 or IL-10 protein to NOD mice, or transgenic expression of the IL-4 (but not IL-10) gene in their islets, prevents insulitis and diabetes.[19,20,133,134] In accordance with this, IL-4 or IL-10 gene therapies, which promote Th2 activity, ameliorate this disease (Table 3). IL-10 is discussed separately in another section below. We compared the effects of delivering IL-4 with an IL-4/IgG1-Fc fusion gene, or inhibiting IFNγ with an IFNγR/IgG1-Fc fusion gene (this vector is described below).[4] The positive effects of the soluble FNγ receptor were significant but less than IL-4/IgG1-Fc, and are described separately. Following i.m. delivery of the IL-4/IgG1-Fc vector serum levels were low (< 10 pg/ml), compared to other vectors we have tested. Nevertheless, IL-4/IgG1-Fc was potently active in vivo, consistent with other observations that this cytokine is immunomodulatory even at very low circulating levels.[135] As in the case of TGF-β1 gene therapy, NOD mice injected with the IL-4/IgG1-Fc plasmid were protected from inflammatory pancreatic-islet lesions and had a much lower incidence of diabetes.[4] Other authors have reported similar protective effects of the IL-4 gene after epidermal gene-gun delivery of a plasmid[136] or systemic adenoviral injections.[137] Interestingly, protein administration in NOD mice must be started as early as 2 weeks of age to prevent diabetes, although we found that gene transfer of IL-4 was effective when started later.

We also examined the effects of TGF-β1 and IL-4/IgG1-Fc cDNA transfer in murine EAE.[3] I.m. TGF-β1 plasmid delivery had pronounced downregulatory effects on T cell proliferation and production of IFNγ and TNFα, on in vitro restimulation with MBP. IL-4/IgG1-Fc vector administration also suppressed these responses, although much less than TGF-β1, and enhanced secretion of endogenous IL-4. Therapy resulted in a significant decrease in the severity of histopathologic inflammatory lesions. In the CNS, treatment with either vector suppressed IL-12 and IFNγ mRNA expression, while IL-4 and TGF-β1 mRNA levels were increased compared with control mice. Thus, cytokine plasmid treatment appeared to inhibit MBP-specific pathogenic Thl responses, while enhancing endogenous secretion of protective cytokines. We demonstrated that gene therapy with these vectors is an effective therapeutic strategy for EAE.

Croxford and coworkers[138] recently reported that i.m. injection of plasmids encoding TGF-β1 and IL-4 failed to influence the clinical course of EAE. This discrepancy with our results may be due to the fact that no detectable plasmid-derived cytokine production was observed in their experiments. Furthermore, they administered plasmid DNA as a single dose in tibialis anterior muscles concurrently with MBP immunization. In our study, plasmid DNA was administered 48 hours before both the initial MBP priming and recall immunizations. Furthermore, we used a plasmid vector, VR1255, selected for high expression in skeletal muscle, and clearly superior for this purpose compared to most other vectors described in the literature. Nevertheless, Croxford et al[138] observed that EAE was ameliorated by a single injection of therapeutic cytokine (IL-4, IFNβ, or TGF-β) plasmid DNA-cationic liposome complex directly into the CNS. DNA coding for a dimeric form of human p75 TNF receptor also improved the disease. This clearly demonstrates that tissue-specific expression of immune mediators relevant to an autoimmune disease can be accomplished with plasmid vectors.

IL-10 Gene Therapy for the Treatment of Inflammatory Diseases

IL-10 has many immunosuppressive and anti-inflammatory effects that could potentially block the autoimmune process at multiple steps.[139-146] Indeed, IL-10 reduces MHC and B7.1/B7.2 expression on APCs, induces T-cell anergy, promotes the differentiation of regulatory T cells (Tr1 type, see below), can increase T-cell apoptosis and can potently suppress pro-inflammatory cytokine expression/function, most notably IFNγ and TNF-α. It has suppressive effects on macrophages and DCs, inhibiting their maturation and consequential ability to promote $CD4^+$ and $CD8^+$ T cell responses. Thus, augmenting IL-10 production in vivo for the purpose of attenuating inflammatory responses and possibly inducing tolerance to autoantigens has been an area of intense scientific investigation.

In recent years, several gene therapy approaches have been developed for IL-10 therapy of inflammatory disorders (Table 3). For instance, systemic delivery of IL-10 by i.m. injection of a plasmid vector prevented autoimmune diabetes in NOD mice.[147] In this case, IL-10 was detectable by ELISA in sera for more than two weeks after injection, and the incidence of diabetes was markedly curtailed. Interestingly, IL-10 did not prevent insulitis, and it appeared that the main effect of therapy was to skew the differentiation of T cells towards the Th2 pathway, consequently inhibiting diabetogenic Th1 cells. In light of more recent studies, however, we hypothesize that this cytokine also acted by inducing Tr1 differentiation. In contrast to this study, the intravenous injection of an IL-10 plasmid complexed to a degradable polymeric carrier, poly[α-(4-aminobutyl)-L-glycolic acid] (PAGA), did ameliorate insulitis.[148] Codelivery of IL-4 and IL-10 cDNA by this method (plasmid/PAGA carrier) also protected against insulitis and diabetes, and proved therapeutically superior to injection of either gene alone.[149,150] In multiple low-dose streptozotocin (STZ)-induced diabetes (MDSD), i.m. delivery of an IL-10 plasmid also protected against insulitis and diabetes.[151] Serum IFNγ levels were reduced, consistent with the pathogenic role of this cytokine in this form of diabetes.

In rat or mouse experimental autoimmune myocarditis, i.m. IL-10 or vIL-10-IgG-Fc gene transfer were both found to be protective.[152-154] For instance, Lewis rats immunized with pig myosin to induce myocarditis were treated with an IL-10 plasmid, transferred into the tibialis anterior muscles by electroporation.[152] With repeated DNA injections, the serum IL-10 levels were increased to > 250 pg/ml, and treated animal had significantly reduced myocardial inflammatory lesions and prolonged survival. Other investigators showed that injection of a plasmid carrying the fusion of vIL-10 with an immunoglobulin Fc fragment resulted in much higher circulating levels of protein (up to 195 ng/ml), which protected against mouse viral myocarditis.[154]

In a murine experimental autoimmune thyroiditis model, direct injection of an IL-10 plasmid into the thyroid gland considerably reduced the lymphocytic infiltration.[155] Similarly, other authors[156] delivered an IL-10 plasmid complexed to a mixture of liposomes and poly-L-Lysine to enhance transfection. There was a significant diminution in the proliferative T-cell response to thyroglobulin (the target antigen) and lower production of IFNγ or Th2 bias in the response. These studies demonstrate that nonviral IL-10 gene therapy can be applied in a tissue-localized fashion.

Inflammatory bowel diseases (IBD), including Crohn's disease and ulcerative colitis are chronic inflammatory disorders of the gastrointestinal tract where initiation and aggravation of the inflammatory process seem to be due to a massive local mucosal immune response where IL-10 correlates with protection.[157,158] Multiple strategies of IL-10 treatment for IBD have been described and include systemic administration of recombinant IL-10, the use of genetically modified bacteria, gelatine microspheres containing IL-10, adenoviral vectors encoding IL-10 and IL-10-secreting regulatory T cells (see below).[157] Although most results of recombinant IL-10 therapies are disappointing in clinical testing because of low efficacy or side effects, therapeutic strategies utilizing gene therapy may enhance mucosal delivery and increase the therapeutic response. Novel IL-10-related cytokines, including IL-19, IL-20, IL-22, IL-24, IL-26, IL-28 and IL-29, are involved in regulation of inflammatory immune responses. Thus, the use of IL-10 and IL-10-related cytokines may provide new insights into future cell-based and gene-based treatments against chronic inflammatory diseases like IBD.

Cytokine Gene Therapy and the Induction of Regulatory T Cells (Tr)

The use of cytokine gene therapy for the treatment and/or establishment of tolerance in chronic inflammatory conditions is expectedly associated with a state of reduced immunoreactivity to self-tissues. Investigators very often infer the existence of an induced/expanded regulatory T cell population underlying this state of hyporesposiveness, although regulation of T cell responses can readily occur in the functional absence of regulatory T cells. Indeed, the negative regulation of innate and adaptive immunity is highly complex, occurring at multiple levels through many disparate mechanisms.[159] Nonetheless, the potential of inducing and selectively engaging specific peripheral immunoregulatory networks by means of innovative gene therapy strategies truly represents a novel and critical area of immunotherapy.

What are regulatory T cells and what is their therapeutic benefit? In an attempt to fine-tune and diversify its ability to control adaptive immune responses in a timely and efficient manner, the immune system has evolved numerous mechanisms, including Tr cells, to modulate and down-regulate immune responses at various locations and in various immune settings (Fig. 1).[160,161] To this end, a network of Tr exists to assure T cell immunoregulation at multiple levels depending on the inflammatory burden and anatomical location. Indeed, a large number of Tr cell populations have been described, and for the most part, their definition has been based on their phenotype and, their relative cytokine production capabilities. In general, most of the described Tr cells arise after deliberate antigen exposure and include regulatory Th2 cells (which suppress Th1 associated responses), Th1 cells (which suppress Th2-cell-mediated responses), IL-10-producing Tr1 cells (a subset of IL-10-dependent, antigen-specific regulatory T cells), TGF-β1-secreting Th3 cells, $CD8^+$, natural killer T (NKT), and γδ T cells.

More recently, naturally-occuring $CD4^+CD25^+$ Tr cells, which exist in the unperturbed T cell repertoire and do not arise from experimental immunostimulation, have emerged as a dominant T cell population capable of mediating peripheral tolerance to autoantigens, but whose functions have now been extended to include the regulation of T cell responses directed

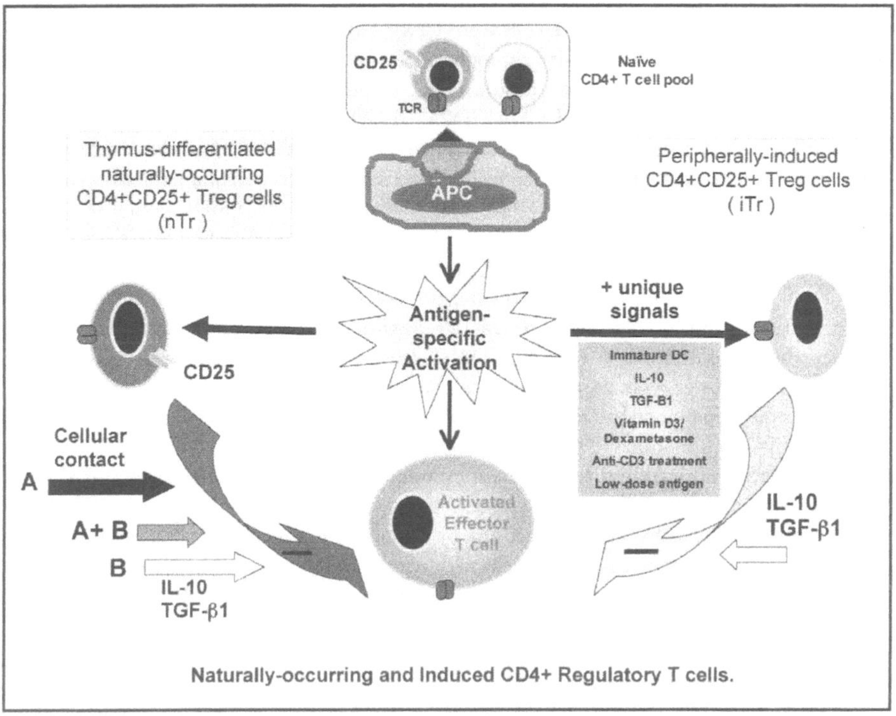

Figure 1. Differentiation pathways of Tr cells. Natural and induced (adaptive) Tr cells arise through different pathways. While the natural Tr cells appear to differentiate in the thymus, the induced Tr cells develop in response to antigenic stimulation and are dependent, at least in part, on cytokines such as TGF-β1 and IL-10 for both their differentiation and suppressive activity.

to foreign antigens. A seminal observation made by Sakaguchi and coworkers,[162] and subsequent work,[163,164] demonstrated that adoptive transfer of $CD4^+CD25^+$-depleted T cells induced several organ-specific autoimmune diseases in recipient, immunodeficient animals, including gastritis, diabetes, IBD, and thyroiditis. Furthermore, cotransfer of these cells with enriched $CD4^+CD25^+$ cells prevented autoimmunity, confirming the regulatory activity of the latter. These findings explained earlier studies, performed 4 decades earlier, which showed that day 3 thymectomy of select strains of neonatal mice disrupted Tr cell development and consequently lead to systemic autoimmunity. $CD4^+CD25^+$ Tr cells consitute 5-10% of $CD4^+$ T cells in mice and humans, and their removal from peripheral immune systems also increases immunity to tumors and allografts. In addition to regulating self-responses, $CD4^+CD25^+$ Tr cells also control immunity to bacterial, fungal, protozoal, nematodal, and viral pathogens.

Several cytokines including IL-10 and TGF-β1, have been implicated in Tr effector functions,[103,141,165,166] and their relative contribution to the generation and effector function of Tr cells remains incompletely defined. While the requirement of cytokines via which Tr cells regulate T responses in vivo are largely determined by tissue- or context-dependent factors, the consensus view is that in vitro $CD4^+CD25^+$ Tr-mediated suppression adopts a contact-dependent, cytokine-independent mechanism of suppression.

The specific generational/stimulatory signals required for the selective expansion and survival in the periphery, particularly in autoimmune -prone subjects, is ill-defined. Failure to obtain compelling answers results, in part, from the fact that different experimental systems are often used, or largely from the fact that investigators routinely fail to discriminate naturally-occurring $CD4^+CD25^+$ T cells from CD25-expressing $CD4^+$ T cell populations induced to acquire suppressor activity throughout the course of an immune response or as a result from a unique stimulatory condition. Thus, the bulk of current literature indicates that there are two general categories of $CD4^+CD25^+$ Tr cells (although there may be subtypes), which differ in their origin and effector mechanism. One Tr subset develops during the normal process of T cell maturation in the thymus, resulting in the generation of a naturally-occurring population of $CD4^+CD25^+$ Tr (nTr) cells that survives in the periphery poised to prevent potential autoimmune responses.[160,161,164] The second subset of induced $CD4^+CD25^+$ Tr (iTr) cells whose precursor is thymically-derived, develops as a consequence of activation of classical naive T cell populations under particular conditions of antigen exposure, cytokine stimulation and/or costimulation.[141,165,166] Thus, $CD4^+$ T cells with regulatory function can be generated by the activation of mature, peripheral $CD4^+$ T cells, and regulatory and pathogenic T cells can, in principle, be generated from the same mature T cell precursors, depending on qualitative and/or quantitative differences in antigen priming. Induced Tr cells can be generated in vivo or ex vivo from mature $CD4^+$CD25- T cell populations under different stimulatory conditions including, antigen in the presence of immunosuppressive cytokines, such as IL-10 and TGF-β1, vitamin D3 and dexamethasone, CD40-CD40L blockade or immature DC populations. It must be noted that antigen exposure by intranasal, intradermal or oral route, seems to selectively induce the appearance of T cells with regulatory phenotype (Th3), whose function in vitro and in vivo generally occurs in a cytokine-dependent manner.[103] Although distinct in nature, it is conceivable that peripheral T cell immunoregulation is assured by a functional synchrony between nTr cell and iTr cell subsets in order to control the activation and function of normal and autoimmune responses.

The relevance of IL-10 to Tr cell differentiation and function has received increasing attention in recent years.[141,160,161,165-167] Although most investigators performing IL-10 gene therapy have not examined this question, a recent study provides interesting information. In accord with previous studies with other vectors, Goudy et al[167] found that systemic treatment of NOD mice with high doses of recombinant adeno-associated virus (rAAV) vector expressing murine IL-10 reduced the severity of insulitis and completely prevented diabetes in all NOD mice, including older 12-week-old mice that are known to resist most forms of immunotherapy. Notably, IL-10 gene therapy dramatically increased the percentage of CD25-expressing $CD4^+$ regulatory T cells, although the cellular origin and functional nature of these cells remains to be defined. Thus, IL-10 treatment of inflammatory conditions may potentially support, under certain circumstances, the induction of $CD4^+$ Tr cells, which can control inflammation.

More recent evidence also suggests that T cell priming in the presence of TGF-β1 potently induces lymphocytes with regulatory potential, suggesting a possible alternate pathway for generating Tr cells in the periphery, as mentioned above.[104-109] Thus, TGF-β1 was shown to induce Foxp3 expression and subsequent regulatory function in murine $CD4^+$CD25- T cells in an IL-2-dependent fashion.[108] Surprisingly, the induced Tr cells appeared to mediate their function in contact-dependent, and cytokine-independent fashion. In a related study, Peng et al[167] showed that transient pulses of TGF-β1 in the islets during the priming phase of diabetes is sufficient to inhibit disease onset by promoting the cycling, expansion and activity of intra-islet $CD4^+CD25^+$ Tr cells which demonstrated features reminiscent of nTr cells: CD25, CTLA-4, and Foxp3 expression. Furthermore, adoptive transfer of these cells potently protected against diabetes. These findings indicate that TGF-β treatment may inhibit autoimmune diseases via the in situ induction, expansion and function of $CD4^+CD25^+$ Tr cells in vivo, thus providing a possible cellular mechanism by which TGF-β can promote immunosuppression and tolerance. Once again, the precise generational and functional relationship of these cells with naturally-occurring Tr cells remains to be defined.

Retroviral Transduction of T Cells and Adoptive Cell Therapy of Autoimmune Disease

Autoimmune disorders represent inappropriate immune responses directed at self-tissue. Antigen-specific $CD4^+$ T cells and antigen-presenting dendritic cells (DCs) are important mediators in the pathogenesis of autoimmune disease and thus are ideal candidates for adoptive cellular gene therapy, an ex vivo approach to therapeutic gene transfer. As discussed in another chapter, retrovirally transduced primary T cells rapidly and preferentially home to the sites of inflammation in animal models of multiple sclerosis, arthritis, and diabetes. These cells, transduced with retroviral vectors to drive expression of various regulatory cytokines such as IL-4, IL-10, and IL-12p40 antagonists, deliver these immunoregulatory proteins to the inflamed lesions, providing therapy for autoimmune diseases.

Gene Therapy of Lupus with Cytokine Inhibitors

Cytokine inhibitors (usually antibodies or soluble cytokine receptors) are advantageously nontoxic and often long-lived in body fluids, compared with most cytokines, Most gene therapy studies of cytokine inhibitors have been carried out with viral vectors, and there is less experience with nonviral methods. However, we and others have shown that the plasmid-based transfer of cDNA encoding these molecules protects against several autoimmune diseases (Table 4). As mentioned above, we constructed an expression plasmid encoding an IFNγR/IgG1-Fc fusion protein.[2,4,5] The appropriate murine cDNA segments were inserted into the plasmid VR1255 (Vical Inc., San Diego, CA), which is exceptionally effective in muscle.[37] It has a CMV IE-EP, CMV intron A, and a rabbit beta-globin transcriptional terminator. COS-7 cells transfected with this plasmid secreted IFNγR/IgG1-Fc fusion protein in vitro as a disulfide-linked homodimer, with the expected biological activity.[2] Thus, IFNγR/IgG1-Fc neutralized IFNγ-dependent NO production by macrophages (stimulated with IFNγ and lipopolysaccharide [LPS]). I.m. injections (100 μg naked DNA/muscle into 2 muscles, administered twice) of the IFNγR/IgG1-Fc plasmid in normal mice resulted in IFNγR/IgG1-Fc serum levels exceeding 100 ng/ml for months after treatment. Higher levels (> 200 ng/ml) were produced by repeated DNA injections.

Our studies showed that soluble receptor levels in the range of 100-200 ng/ml effectively blocked IFNγ-induced pathology in four different experimental models. The high-level and long-term expression of this vector, compared with many other plasmid vectors, may be related

Table 4. Examples of plasmid-based anticytokine gene therapy

Inhibitor	Disease	References
IFNγR/IgG-Fc	Multiple dose STZ[1]-induced diabetes	1
	NOD-mouse autoimmune diabetes	4
	Murine lupus	5
TNFα receptors[2]	EAE	138
	Arthritis (CIA)	173-175
IL-1Ra	Arthritis (CIA)	172

1. Abbreviations: CIA, collagen-induced arthritis; EAE, experimental autoimmune encephalomyelitis; IFNγR/IgG-Fc, interferon γ receptor/IgG-Fc fusion protein; IL-1Ra, IL-1 receptor antagonist; STZ, streptozotocin.
2. Soluble chimeric TNF receptors, usually produced as either TNF-receptor/IgG-Fc proteins, or fusion of TNF receptor components.

to the neutralization of IFNγ, since this cytokine can suppress transcription promoted by CMV IE-EP elements.

Many abnormalities in the cytokine network have been reported in lupus, but increased levels of IFNγ, as well as some IFNαβ species, in serum, lymphoid organs and inflamed tissues are prominent.[18,168] In particular, the production of IFNγ is remarkably high in MRL-*lpr/lpr* lupus-prone mice.[5,169] Therefore, it was of interest to determine if IFNγ could be blocked by a gene therapy approach. We inoculated an IFNγR/IgG1-Fc plasmid into lupus-prone and observed low level expression compared with a previous study in NOD and CD1 mice with the same vector. However, serum IFNγ levels of untreated MRL-*lpr/lpr* mice are very high, and it is possible the soluble receptor was removed after binding to IFNγ. Alternatively, residual IFNγ might have shut down the vector's IFNγ-sensitive CMV enhancer/promoter.

When in vivo electroporation was applied to enhance gene transfer in MRL *lpr/lpr* mice, serum IFNγR/IgG1-Fc levels, which had been < 10 ng/ml without electroporation, exceeded 100 ng/ml and, consequently, IFN-γ serum levels were markedly reduced.[5] Thus, electroporation was remarkably effective, and it is likely that this technique will be even more relevant to other species. Indeed, as mentioned previously, in primates and other large mammals i.m. gene transfer of naked DNA is not as efficient as in rodents, but is greatly augmented by in vivo electroporation.

Treatment with the IFN-γR/IgG1 plasmid by i.m. injections, especially with electroporation, protected MRL *lpr/lpr* mice from early death, and reduced autoantibody titres, renal disease and histological markers of SLE-like disease.[5] Most notably, when therapy was initiated in 4 month-old diseased mice, survival was extended beyond expectations, with 100% of the mice staying alive at 14 months of age compared with none in the control group. Remarkably, disease severity was reduced or even suppressed in the treated group.

The mechanism(s) by which IFNγ contributes to the pathogenesis of lupus is not clear, but there are important clues. IFNγ promotes production of autoantibodies of the IgG2a and IgG3 isotypes that efficiently activate complement. In addition, IgG3 has cryogenic properties. Furthermore, IFNγ enhances several pathogenic activities of macrophages and promotes inflammation in target tissues.

Other investigators have attempted to neutralize IFNγ in mouse lupus models using polyclonal and monoclonal antibodies (mAbs), as well as soluble IFNγR. These approaches, however, have limitations. For example, large quantities of mAbs would be required and may not achieve sufficient concentration in tissues to be effective, and/or they may be neutralized by the host immune response. With regard to soluble recombinant receptors, rapid turnover may affect efficacy and necessitates repeated administration. These constraints possibly explain previous negative results of anti-IFNγ mAb treatment of MRL *lpr/lpr* mice, and the finding that treatment with recombinant soluble IFNγR in NZBxNZWF1 lupus mice was effective only when initiated early, but not late, when IFNγ levels are significantly higher.[170]

The IFNγR/IgG1-Fc fusion protein produced in these studies is comprised of segments of endogenous murine proteins. Antibodies reactive with these proteins do not appear to be produced in treated mice, even after repeated injections of plasmid over several weeks. In this respect, it now clear that plasmids that do not encode immunogenic proteins, or plasmids injected into immunodeficient SCID mice, are expressed for longer periods. This may be related to the fact that myocytes encoding xenogeneic proteins can be attacked and killed by the immune system, as observed in DNA vaccination studies, and/or because locally produced IFNγ or other cytokines inhibit vector expression.

The addition of an Fc segment to a therapeutic protein is not always essential, but may confer significant advantages. The Fc portion simplifies purification of the recombinant protein by affinity chromatography, and the increase in size can prolong the half-life of small proteins in body fluids. For instance, the half-life of the truncated IFNγ receptor is quite short compared with a receptor/Fc fusion protein.[171] Also, dimers are likely to have a higher avidity for their ligand, as is clearly the case with the IFNγ receptor.

Cytokine Inhibitors in Arthritis

IL-1Ra is an endogenous protein that can prevent the binding of IL-1 to its cell-surface receptors. IL-1Ra has shown promise in the therapy of arthritis, and is a candidate molecule for gene therapy. However, almost all studies have been conducted with viral vectors. Recently, Kim et al[172] investigated i.m. plasmid-based IL-1ra therapy in the prevention of murine collagen-induced arthritis (CIA). In bovine type II collagen-immunized DBA/1 mice, delivery of IL-1ra cDNA significantly reduced joint pathology. Synovitis and cartilage erosion in knee joints were markedly reduced, and the expression of IL-1β was significantly decreased in the ankle joints of mice treated with IL-1Ra. This occurred despite the fact that the levels of IL-1Ra in sera and joints after i.m. injection of IL-1Ra DNA were significantly lower than when protein had been used in previous reports.

Kim and colleagues,[173] Bloquel et al[174] and Gould et al[175] have also reported on the effectiveness of plasmid-based transfer of soluble TNF-receptor cDNA in CIA, as described in another chapter. As expected, in vivo electroporation increases the effectiveness of these vectors. In one study, the inhibition of established CIA was performed with a doxycycline regulated plasmid.[175] Protection against CIA has also been achieved by transfer of IL-4[176] and IL-10.[177,178] These studies demonstrate that nonviral gene therapy can be effective against arthritis, at least when gene transfer is enhanced by electroporation.

Cytokine Inhibitors in Other Autoimmune Diseases

The transfer of cDNA encoding cytokine inhibitors protects against several autoimmune diseases (Table 4). IL-12 and IFNγ are usually detrimental in autoimmune diseases and, consequently, their neutralization is likely to be protective. These two cytokines are functionally related, since IL-12 induces IFNγ production by T cells and NK cells, while IFNγ mediates or augments many of the effects initiated by IL-12. The neutralization of IFNγ with mAbs or soluble receptors prevents NOD-mouse diabetes,[2,8,9,179] as well as diabetes induced by administration of multiple low-dose STZ (MDSD) in other strains.[171] CYP greatly accelerates disease in NOD mice, and the CYP- and STZ-induced diseases are both associated with a burst of systemic and intra-islet IFNγ release.[180] Indeed, we observed that i.m. administration of an IFNγ expression plasmid accelerated disease in NOD mice,[1] and others found that nondiabetes-prone transgenic mice expressing IFNγ in their islets developed insulitis/diabetes associated with a loss of tolerance to islet antigens.[181] IFNγ, IL-12, IL-18 and other inflammatory cytokines are produced locally in the inflamed islets of NOD mice.[19,20] Furthermore, microarray analysis of the islets of CYP-treated mice revealed that IFNγ dominated the changes in gene expression to a striking degree.[182] Surprisingly, gene expression related to Tr cells was not markedly altered. IFNγ is toxic to islet cells, particularly in combination with IL-1 and TNFα(reviewed in refs. 19,20). Also, it could act by activating macrophages, stimulating Th1 cells, or augmenting CTL and NK activity. All these cells have the potential to injure or kill islet cells.

In vivo, administration of our IFNγR/IgG1-Fc vector almost completely blocked the systemic IFNγ activity induced by either STZ (CD-1 or C57BL/6 mice) or CYP (NOD mice).[2] Moreover, this plasmid was protective in either natural or drug-induced models of autoimmune diabetes,[2,4] in agreement with the postulated pathogenic role of IFNγ. In each case, therapy reduced the severity insulitis and the frequency of diabetes which is secondary to this lesion. It should be noted, however, that this anti-cytokine therapy was more effective in the induced models of diabetes (STZ of CYP), presumably because IFNγ plays a more important role in the pathogenesis of these diseases. Nevertheless, IFNγR/IgG1-Fc gene therapy protected NOD mice and, interestingly, this was superior to IFNγ gene knockout which has only a modest effect.[183] The reason is unclear, but mice deficient in IFNγ from fetal life may develop compensatory mechanisms.

RNA Interference with Nonviral Vectors

It is now well established that double-stranded RNA (dsRNA) induces gene silencing in a sequence specific way.[184-187] Double-stranded siRNAs (short inhibitory RNAs) are produced from dsRNA through the activity of an RNase III family endonuclease denoted Dicer.[184-187] They are generally 21 to 23 nucleotide long and have overhanging ends consisting of two nucleotides. siRNAs interact with a large multi-component enzyme termed RNA-induced silencing complex (RISC), to bind a fully complementary mRNA sequence, which results in endonucleolytic cleavage of the mRNA. RISC has two key components, i.e., siRNAs and Argonaute family proteins, and it is the Argonaute2 protein that actually cuts the mRNA.[188] The cleaved RNA is further degraded by cellular exonuclease activities. siRNAs provide a stronger method of gene silencing than either antisense molecules or ribozymes. They are short enough to avoid induction of an interferon response, and this increases their research applicability and therapeutic potential immensely. Indeed, several in vivo applications have already been reported (Table 1).

Other types of short RNAs have equally impressive gene silencing properties.[187,189] Diverse eukaryotic species, including humans, possess noncoding regulatory endogenous hairpin RNAs (microRNAs [miRNA]), that can interact with RISC and silence genes. However, unlike siRNAs, miRNAs do not induce degradation of mRNA, but rather partially bind to its 3' UTR and block translation.[187,189] Thus, RISC can interfere with protein synthesis and this is the dominant mechanisms used by miRNAs in mammals. In addition, short RNAs can shut down gene expression by inducing specific methylation of promoters, in several species including humans.[190]

It is reasonably simple to deliver siRNAs to cells in vitro, with methods such as cationic lipids or electroporation, but delivery in vivo is more difficult. For in vivo administration, hydrodynamic delivery and electroporation have both been employed. For example, McCaffrey et al[191] and Lewis et al[192] silenced genes in vivo in mice by injecting siRNA in the tail vein under pressure. Liver uptake of siRNA was observed, and a sequence-specific gene silencing effect in that organ persisted for 3 or 4 days. Other studies showed that the intravenous injection of Fas-specific siRNA protected against hepatitis and hepatic necrosis induced by administration of either concanavalin A (Con A) or anti-Fas monoclonal antibodies.[193] Caspase 8 siRNA also protected against acute liver failure in similar models.[194] Remarkably, improved survival due to caspase 8 RNA interference was observed when treatment was applied during ongoing acute liver failure. A limitation of these methods is that the siRNA is distributed to multiple organs.

Hagstrom et al[195] demonstrated delivery of plasmid DNA or siRNA by injection into the distal veins of limbs transiently isolated from the circulation by a tourniquet. Delivery to myocytes was facilitated by the rapid injection of sufficient volume to permit extravasation of the nucleic acid solution into muscle tissue. With this method, they reported siRNA-mediated gene silencing in rat and primate limb muscle. Kishida et al[196] delivered siRNA duplexes corresponding to reporter genes by electroporation into the tibial muscle of mice expressing these reporter genes (transgenic or vector induced). As little as 0.05 μg of siRNA almost completely blocked the expression of a reporter gene from 10 μg of plasmid DNA, for at least one week. In transgenic mice, green fluorescent protein expression was also effectively blocked in cells receiving the complementary siRNA.

Some disadvantages of these methods include the high cost of producing sufficient quantities of siRNA, transient in vivo activity and, in some cases, distribution of the siRNA to tissues outside the target area. These limitations can be circumvented by the administration of siRNA plasmid or viral (adenoviral, retroviral or lentiviral) vectors.[185-187,197,198] Viral vectors, however, are limited by the biological effects they produce, and nonviral methods are often preferable. Furthermore, nonviral methods can be adapted for both systemic and tissue-specific delivery. For example, target tissues have included tumors or limb muscle. Most of these vectors advantageously employ Pol III promoters such as U6, tRNA or H1, although Pol II constructs are feasible.[187] Various designs are possible,[187] e.g., vectors producing two separate complementary RNA strands, or producing short hairpin RNAs (shRNAs). The shRNAs are processed in vivo by Dicer, to generate active siRNAs. The vector can also produce a modified miRNA that is also processed by Dicer. The use of plasmid or viral vectors allows the introduction of tissue-specific or drug-sensitive promoters, to either limit expression to a target tissue or limit expression to a desired period of time.

The applications of siRNA technology are numerous. It represents a powerful research tool for studying physiological and pathological gene function.[184-187] The in vitro or in vivo delivery of siRNA of obvious interest for investigative or therapeutic purposes in infectious and inflammatory diseases, as well as cancer.[186,187,191-198] Indeed, its therapeutic potential has been clearly demonstrated in murine models of viral hepatitis, where both synthetic and plasmid-based siRNA therapy has been effective in suppressing the expression of viruses.[199] Electroporation-enhanced plasmid siRNA delivery, with appropriate modifications, should be applicable to many tissues.

Nonviral Gene Transfer in Humans

There have been questions as to whether nonviral gene therapy and/or DNA vaccination are effective in large mammals. However, plasmid-based gene transfer for DNA vaccination or other purposes has been successfully performed in pigs, dogs, ruminants, horses, nonhuman primates and humans.[200,201] Therapeutic levels of angiogenic factors have been generated in human skeletal and cardiac muscle.[202,203] Of note, in the future, gene transfer could be greatly improved by introducing electroporation, hydrodynamic delivery or other new approaches. Nonviral gene transfer is particularly applicable to cancer therapy. For instance, some authors have investigated gene therapy for malignant gliomas by in vivo transduction with the human IFNβ gene using cationic liposomes,[208] and other clinical trials are ongoing.

Most of the human studies have been in the area of DNA vaccination. Notably, immune responses can be generated against malaria antigens by i.m. DNA vaccination, and recent studies point to heterologous plasmid/virus prime-boost strategies as an effective method of generating immunity.[204-207] Antigen-reactive T cells are readily induced, but antibody responses are usually of low magnitude. Vaccination is well tolerated, with either few or no side effects. In fact, nonviral DNA transfer into humans has had a remarkable safety profile, and is attracting more attention for this reason. Therefore, there is no obvious contra-indication for the use of these techniques in patients with autoimmune disease.

Conclusions and Future Prospects

The gene therapy of autoimmune diseases holds great promise. Unlike protein therapy, it allows long-term and relatively constant delivery of many cytokines or cytokine inhibitors at therapeutic levels even after one or a few treatments. Moreover, organ-specific delivery of mediators is feasible, either by direct injection of vectors into tissues or, as discussed in other chapters, by ex vivo transduction of cells, which can be reimplanted. Autoreactive T cells can also be transduced ex vivo, and transferred into recipients where they home to target tissues.

Viral and nonviral vectors have been used to protect against organ-specific and systemic autoimmune diseases in several models. TGF-β1 gene therapy protects against murine lupus, autoimmune diabetes, EAE, arthritis and colitis. IL-4 and IL-10 have also proved effective in several autoimmune conditions.

In our laboratories, we relied on administration of plasmid DNA into skeletal muscle. These vectors are nonimmunogenic and can be expressed in muscle for months. Naked DNA injection usually generates relatively low levels of circulating cytokines, which can often be advantageous, since these mediators are active at very low levels, while high levels can be severely toxic. When higher levels of expression are desired, as with cytokine inhibitors, this can be accomplished by applying in vivo electroporation.

The delivery of inhibitory soluble cytokine receptors, or other cytokine inhibitors, has significant advantages over other methods. The neutralization of IFNγ and IL-1 is particularly effective in models of lupus and arthritis, respectively. These receptors have no direct toxic or adverse effects other than depressed immunity, but only as related to the neutralization of one cytokine. Most, if not all, immunosuppressive drugs have many adverse effects and much broader suppressive activity. Cytokines can be blocked with monoclonal antibodies, but even humanized immunoglobulins can give rise to a neutralizing immune response in the recipient. In contrast, soluble receptors made only of self elements are much less likely to be neutralized.

The use of nonviral nucleic acids in experimental therapy is constantly expanding. This includes the application of CpG ODNs to the immunotherapy of cancer and allergic diseases. The most remarkable new development, however, is the introduction of siRNA-based therapeutic agents. Indeed, synthetic or vector-delivered siRNAs are powerful new tools for gene silencing, and their potential therapeutic applications are numerous. However, targeting the in vivo delivery of these molecules to a specific tissue is difficult, and nonviral methods of nucleic acid transfer, such as electroporation or hydronamic delivery, have advantages in terms of simplicity, effectiveness and safety.

Many tools are now available to the immunologist, at least experimentally, to treat inflammatory diseases, but few are as promising as the gene therapy or other nucleic acid transfer approaches.

Acknowledgements

Our studies were funded by the Juvenile Diabetes Research Foundation, the Canadian Diabetes Association, the National Cancer Institute of Canada, the Canadian Institutes of Health Research, the St. Michael's Hospital Foundation, and the National Institutes of Health (USA; grants AR31203, AG15061, and AR39555). We thank Vical Inc. (San Diego, California) for providing the VR1255 expression plasmid used in our studies.

References

1. Piccirillo CA, Chang Y, Prud'homme GJ. Transforming growth factor beta-1 (TGF-β1) somatic gene therapy prevents autoimmune disease in NOD mice. J Immunol 1998; 161:3950-3956.
2. Prud'homme GJ, Chang Y. Prevention of autoimmune diabetes by intramuscular gene therapy with a nonviral vector encoding an interferon-gamma receptor/IgG1 fusion protein. Gene Ther 1999; 6:771-777.
3. Piccirillo CA, Prud'homme GJ. Prevention of experimental allergic encephalomyelitis by intramuscular gene transfer with cytokine-encoding plasmid vectors. Hum Gene Ther 1999; 10:1915-1922.
4. Chang Y, Prud'homme GJ. Intramuscular administration of expression plasmids encoding interferon-gamma-receptor/IgG1 or IL-4/IgG1 chimeric proteins protects from autoimmunity. J Gene Med 1999; 1:415-423.
5. Lawson BR, Prud'homme GJ, Chang Y et al. Treatment of mouse lupus with cDNA encoding IFN-γR/Fc. J Clin Invest 2000; 106:207-215.

6. Prud'homme GJ, Piccirillo CA. Inhibitory effects of transforming growth factor beta-1 in autoimmune diseases. J Autoimmun 2000; 14:23-42.
7. Prud'homme GJ. Gene therapy of autoimmune diseases with vectors encoding regulatory cytokines or inflammatory cytokine inhibitors. J Gene Med 2000; 2:222-232.
8. Prud'homme GJ, Lawson BR, Chang Y et al. Immunotherapeutic gene transfer into muscle. Trends Immunol 2001; 22:149-155.
9. Prud'homme GJ, Lawson BR, Theofilopoulos AN. Anticytokine gene therapy of autoimmune diseases. Expert Opin Biol Ther 2001; 1:359-373.
10. Piccirillo CA, Prud'homme GJ. Immune modulation by plasmid DNA-mediated cytokine gene transfer. Curr Pharm Des 2003; 9:83-94.
11. Piccirillo CA, Prud'homme GJ. Gene therapy with plasmids encoding cytokine- or cytokine receptor-IgG chimeric proteins. Methods Mol Biol 2003; 215:153-70.
12. Mageed RA, Prud'homme GJ. Immunopathology and gene therapy of lupus. Gene Ther 2003; 10:861-874.
13. Dinarello CA. The IL-1 family and inflammatory diseases. Clin Exp Rheumatol 2002; 20(5 Suppl 27):S1-13.
14. Feldmann M, Brennan FM, Williams RO et al. The transfer of a laboratory based hypothesis to a clinically useful therapy: The development of anti-TNF therapy of rheumatoid arthritis. Best Pract Res Clin Rheumatol 2004; 18:59-80.
15. Vilcek J, Feldmann M. Historical review: Cytokines as therapeutics and targets of therapeutics. Trends Pharmacol Sci 2004; 25:201-209.
16. Feldmann M, Brennan FM, Foxwell BM et al. The role of TNF alpha and IL-1 in rheumatoid arthritis. Curr Dir Autoimmun 2001; 3:188-199.
17. Feldmann M, Maini RN. Anti-TNF alpha therapy of rheumatoid arthritis: What have we learned? Annu Rev Immunol 2001; 19:163-916.
18. Theofilopoulos AN, Lawson BR. Tumour necrosis factor and other cytokines in murine lupus. Ann Rheum Dis 1999; 58(Suppl 1):I49-155.
19. Rabinovitch A, Suarez-Pinzon WL. Role of cytokines in the pathogenesis of autoimmune diabetes mellitus. Rev Endocr Metab Disord 2003; 4:291-299.
20. Rabinovitch A. Immunoregulation by cytokines in autoimmune diabetes. Adv Exp Med Biol 2003; 520:159-193.
21. Vandenbroeck K, Alloza I, Gadina M et al. Inhibiting cytokines of the interleukin-12 family: Recent advances and novel challenges. J Pharm Pharmacol 2004; 56:145-160.
22. Segal BM. Experimental autoimmune encephalomyelitis: Cytokines, effector T cells, and antigen-presenting cells in a prototypical Th1-mediated autoimmune disease. Curr Allergy Asthma Rep 2003; 3:86-93.
23. Lin MT, Pulkkinen L, Uitto J et al. The gene gun: current applications in cutaneous gene therapy. Int J Dermatol 2000; 39:161-170.
24. Furth PA. Gene transfer by biolistic process. Mol Biotechnol 1997; 7:139-143.
25. El-Aneed A. An overview of current delivery systems in cancer gene therapy. J Control Release 2004; 94:1-14.
26. McMahon JM, Wells DJ. Electroporation for gene transfer to skeletal muscles: Current status. Bio Drugs 2004; 18:155-165.
27. Herweijer H, Wolff JA. Progress and prospects: Naked DNA gene transfer and therapy. Gene Ther 2003; 10:453-458.
28. Bigey P, Bureau MF, Scherman D. In vivo plasmid DNA electrotransfer. Curr Opin Biotechnol 2002; 13:443-447.
29. Zhang G, Budker V, Wolff JA. High levels of foreign gene expression in hepatocytes after tail vein injections of naked plasmid DNA. Hum Gene Ther 1999; 10:1735-1737.
30. Zhang G, Budker V, Williams P et al. Efficient expression of naked dna delivered intraarterially to limb muscles of nonhuman primates. Hum Gene Ther 2001; 12:427-438.
31. Hagstrom JE, Hegge J, Zhang G et al. A facile nonviral method for delivering genes and siRNAs to skeletal muscle of mammalian limbs. Mol Ther 2004; 10:386-398.
32. Miller DL, Pislaru SV, Greenleaf JE. Sonoporation: Mechanical DNA delivery by ultrasonic cavitation. Somat Cell Mol Genet 2002; 27:115-134.

33. Hosseinkhani H, Aoyama T, Ogawa O et al. Ultrasound enhances the transfection of plasmid DNA by nonviral vectors. Curr Pharm Biotechnol 2003; 4:109-122.
34. Wells DJ. Gene therapy progress and prospects: Electroporation and other physical methods. Gene Ther 2004; 11:1363-1369.
35. Wolff JA, Malone RW, Williams P et al. Direct gene transfer into mouse muscle in vivo. Science 1990; 247:1465-1468.
36. Wolff JA, Williams P, Acsadi G et al. Conditions affecting direct gene transfer into rodent muscle in vivo. Biotechniques 1991; 11:474-485.
37. Hartikka J, Sawdey M, Cornefert-Jensen F et al. An improved plasmid DNA expression vector for direct injection into skeletal muscle. Hum Gene Ther 1996; 7:1205-1217.
38. Song K, Chang Y, Prud'homme GJ. Regulation of T-helper-1 versus T-helper-2 activity and enhancement of tumor immunity by combined DNA-based vaccination and nonviral cytokine gene transfer. Gene Ther 2000; 7:481-492.
39. Dupuis M, Denis-Mize K, Woo C et al. Distribution of DNA vaccines determines their immunogenicity after intramuscular injection in mice. J Immunol 2000; 165:2850-2858.
40. Muramatsu T, Nakamura A, Park HM. In vivo electroporation: a powerful and convenient means of nonviral gene transfer to tissues of living animals. Int J Mol Med 1998; 1:55-62.
41. Mir LM, Bureau MF, Gehl J et al. High-efficiency gene transfer into skeletal muscle mediated by electric pulses. Proc Natl Acad Sci USA 1999; 96:4262-4267.
42. Lucas Ml, Heller R. Immunomodulation by electrically enhanced delivery of plasmid DNA encoding IL-12 to murine skeletal muscle. Mol Ther 2001; 3:47-53.
43. Mathiesen I. Electropermeabilization of skeletal muscle enhances gene transfer in vivo. Gene Ther 1999; 6:508-514.
44. Rizzuto G, Cappelletti M, Maione D et al. Efficient and regulated erythropoietin production by naked DNA injection and muscle electroporation. Proc Natl Acad Sci USA 1999; 96:6417-6422.
45. Harrison RL, Byrne BJ, Tung L. Electroporation-mediated gene transfer in cardiac tissue. FEBS Letters 1998; 435:1-5.
46. Somiari S, Glasspool-Malone J, Drabick JJ et al. Theory and in vivo application of electroporative gene delivery. Mol Ther 2000; 2:178-187.
47. Bettan M, Emmanuel F, Darteil R et al. High level protein secretion into blood circulation after electric pulse-mediated gene transfer into skeletal muscle. Mol Ther 2000; 2:204-210.
48. Martin JB, Young JL, Benoit Jn et al. Gene transfer to intact mesenteric arteries by electroporation. J Vasc Res 2000; 37:372-380.
49. Dev SB, Rabussay DP, Widera G et al. Medical applications of electroporation. IEEE Transactions on Plasma Science 2000; 28:206-223.
50. Suzuki T, Shin BC, Fujikura K et al. Direct gene transfer into rat liver cells by in vivo electroporation. FEBS Letters 1998; 425:436-440.
51. Nishi T, Yoshizato K, Yamashiro S et al. High-efficiency in vivo gene transfer using intraarterial plasmid DNA injection following in vivo electroporation. Cancer Res 1996; 56:1050-1055.
52. Neumann E, Kakorin S, Toensing K. Fundamentals of electroporative delivery of drugs and genes. Bioelectrochem & Bioenergetics 1999; 48:3-16.
53. Singh BN, Dwivedi C. Antitumor drug delivery by tissue electroporation. Anti-Cancer Drugs 1999; 10:139-146.
54. Zhou ZF, Peretz Y, Chang Y et al. Intramuscular gene transfer of soluble B7.1/IgG(1) fusion cDNA induces potent antitumor immunity as an adjuvant for DNA vaccination. Cancer Gene Ther 2003; 10(6):491-9.
55. Gothelf A, Mir LM, Gehl J. Electrochemotherapy: Results of cancer treatment using enhanced delivery of bleomycin by electroporation. Cancer Treat Rev 2003; 29:371-387.
56. Mir LM. Therapeutic perspectives of in vivo cell electropermeabilization. Bioelectrochemistry 2001; 53:1-10.
57. Heller R, Gilbert R, Jaroszeski MJ. Clinical applications of electrochemotherapy. Adv Drug Deliv Rev 1999; 35:119-129.
58. Kishida T, Asada H, Itokawa Y et al. Electrochemo-gene therapy of cancer: Intratumoral delivery of interleukin-12 gene and bleomycin synergistically induced therapeutic immunity and suppressed subcutaneous and metastatic melanomas in mice. Mol Ther 2003; 8:738-745.

59. Klinman DM. Immunotherapeutic uses of CpG oligodeoxynucleotides. Nat Rev Immunol 2004; 4:249-258.
60. Krieg AM. CpG motifs in bacterial DNA and their immune effects. Annu Rev Immunol 2002; 20:709-760.
61. Vollmer J, Weeratna R, Payette P et al. Characterization of three CpG oligodeoxynucleotide classes with distinct immunostimulatory activities. Eur J Immunol 2004; 34:251-62.
62. Rothenfusser S, Tuma E, Endres S et al. Plasmacytoid dendritic cells: The key to CpG. Hum Immunol 2002; 63:1111-1119.
63. Hochrein H, O'Keeffe M, Wagner H. Human and mouse plasmacytoid dendritic cells. Hum Immunol 2002; 63:1103-1110.
64. Ishii KJ, Gursel I, Gursel M et al. Immunotherapeutic utility of stimulatory and suppressive oligodeoxynucleotides. Curr Opin Mol Ther 2004; 6:166-174.
65. Klinman DM, Zeuner R, Yamada H et al. Regulation of CpG-induced immune activation by suppressive oligodeoxynucleotides. Ann N Y Acad Sci 2003; 1002:112-123.
66. Qin L, Ding Y, Pahud DR et al. Promoter attenuation in gene therapy: Interferon-gamma and tumor necrosis factor-alpha inhibit transgene expression. Hum Gene Ther 1997; 8:2019-2029.
67. Chen D, Murphy B, Sung R et al. Adaptive and innate immune responses to gene transfer vectors: Role of cytokines and chemokines in vector function. Gene Ther 2003; 10:991-998.
68. Bromberg JS, Debruyne LA, Qin L. Interactions between the immune system and gene therapy vectors: Bidirectional regulation of response and expression. Adv Immunol 1998; 69:353-409.
69. Reyes-Sandoval A, Ertl HC. CpG methylation of a plasmid vector results in extended transgene product expression by circumventing induction of immune responses. Mol Ther 2004; 9:249-261.
70. Chen ZY, He CY, Ehrhardt A et al. Minicircle DNA vectors devoid of bacterial DNA result in persistent and high-level transgene expression in vivo. Mol Ther 2003; 8:495-500.
71. Darquet AM, Rangara R, Kreiss P et al. Minicircle: An improved DNA molecule for in vitro and in vivo gene transfer. Gene Ther 1999; 6:209-218.
72. Pasare C, Medzhitov R. Toll pathway-dependent blockade of $CD4^{+}CD25^{+}$ T cell-mediated suppression by dendritic cells. Science 2003; 299:1033-1036.
73. Horner AA, Raz E. DNA-based immunotherapeutics for allergic disease. In: Raz E, ed. Microbial DNA and Host Immunity. Humana Press, 2002:279-299.
74. Kitigaki K, Kline JN. CpG oligodeoxynucleotides in asthma. In: Raz E, ed. Microbial DNA and Host Immunity. Humana Press, 2002:301-314.
75. Keane-Myers A, Chan CC. Modulation of allergic conjunctivitis by immunostimulatory DNA sequence oligonucleotides. In: Raz E, ed. Microbial DNA and Host Immunity. Humana Press, 2002:315-325.
76. Jain VV, Kline JN. CpG DNA: Immunomodulation and remodelling of the asthmatic airway. Expert Opin Biol Ther 2004; 4:1533-1540.
77. Jain VV, Kitagaki K, Kline JN. CpG DNA and immunotherapy of allergic airway diseases. Clin Exp Allergy 2003; 33:1330-1335.
78. Jain VV, Kitagaki K, Businga T et al. CpG-oligodeoxynucleotides inhibit airway remodeling in a murine model of chronic asthma. J Allergy Clin Immunol 2002; 110:867-872.
79. Shirota H, Sano K, Kikuchi T et al. Regulation of murine airway eosinophilia and Th2 cells by antigen-conjugated CpG oligodeoxynucleotides as a novel antigen-specific immunomodulator. J Immunol 2000; 164:5575-5582.
80. Datta SK, Cho HJ, Takabayashi K et al. Antigen-immunostimulatory oligonucleotide conjugates: Mechanisms and applications. Immunol Rev 2004; 199:217-226.
81. Datta SK, Takabayashi K, Raz E. The therapeutic potential of antigen-oligonucleotide conjugates. Ann NY Acad Sci 2003; 1002:105-111.
82. Kitagaki K, Jain VV, Businga TR et al. Immunomodulatory effects of CpG oligodeoxynucleotides on established th2 responses. Clin Diagn Lab Immunol 2002; 9:1260-1269.
83. Davis HL, Millan CL, Watkins SC. Immune-mediated destruction of transfected muscle fibers after direct gene transfer with antigen-expressing plasmid DNA. Gene Ther 1997; 4:181-188.
84. Rui L, Vinuesa CG, Blasioli J et al. Resistance to CpG DNA-induced autoimmunity through tolerogenic B cell antigen receptor ERK signaling. Nat Immunol 2003; 4:594-600.

85. Tran TT, Reich 3rd CF, Alam M et al. Specificity and immunochemical properties of anti-DNA antibodies induced in normal mice by immunization with mammalian DNA with a CpG oligonucleotide as adjuvant. Clin Immunol 2003; 109:278-287.
86. Pizetsky DS. The antigenic properties of bacterial DNA in normal and aberrant immunity. Springer Semin Immunopathol 2000; 22:153-166.
87. Gilkeson GS, Ruiz P, Pippen AM et al. Modulation of renal disease in autoimmune NZB/NZW mice by immunization with bacterial DNA. J Exp Med 1996; 183:1389-1397.
88. Anders HJ, Vielhauer V, Eis V et al. Activation of toll-like receptor-9 induces progression of renal disease in MRL-Fas(lpr) mice. FASEB J 2004; 18:534-536.
89. Hasegawa K, Hayashi T et al. Synthetic CpG oligodeoxynucleotides accelerate the development of lupus nephritis during preactive phase in NZB x NZWF1 mice. Lupus 2003; 12:838-845.
90. Zeuner RA, Verthelyi D, Gursel M et al. Influence of stimulatory and suppressive DNA motifs on host susceptibility to inflammatory arthritis. Arthritis Rheum 2003; 48:1701-1707.
91. Zeuner RA, Ishii KJ, Lizak MJ et al. Reduction of CpG-induced arthritis by suppressive oligodeoxynucleotides. Arthritis Rheum 2002; 46:2219-2224.
92. Schiller M, Javelaud D, Mauviel A. TGF-beta-induced SMAD signaling and gene regulation: Consequences for extracellular matrix remodeling and wound healing. J Dermatol Sci 2004; 35:83-92.
93. ten Dijke P, Hill CS. New insights into TGF-beta-Smad signalling. Trends Biochem Sci 2004; 29:265-273.
94. Derynck R, Zhang YE. Smad-dependent and Smad-independent pathways in TGF-beta family signalling. Nature 2003; 425:577-584.
95. Wahl SM, Chen W. TGF-beta: How tolerant can it be? Immunol Res 2003; 28:167-179.
96. Wahl SM, Swisher J, McCartney-Francis N et al. TGF-beta: The perpetrator of immune suppression by regulatory T cells and suicidal T cells. J Leukoc Biol 2004; 76:15-24.
97. Luethviksson BR, Gunnlaugsdottir B. Transforming growth factor-beta as a regulator of site-specific T-cell inflammatory response. Scand J Immunol 2003; 58:129-38.
98. Levings MK, Bacchetta R, Schulz U et al. The role of IL-10 and TGF-beta in the differentiation and effector function of T regulatory cells. Int Arch Allergy Immunol 2002; 129:263-276.
99. Leask A, Abraham DJ. TGF-beta signaling and the fibrotic response. FASEB J 2004; 18:816-827.
100. Bommireddy R, Doetschman T. TGF-beta, T-cell tolerance and anti-CD3 therapy. Trends Mol Med 2004; 10:3-9.
101. Siegel PM, Massague J. Cytostatic and apoptotic actions of TGF-beta in homeostasis and cancer. Nat Rev Cancer 2003; 3:807-821.
102. Howe PH. Transforming growth factor beta. In: Thomson AW, Lotze MT, eds. The Cytokine Handbook Fourth Edition. Academic Press, 2003:1119-1152.
103. Wu HY, Weiner HL. Oral tolerance. Immunol Res 2003; 28:265-284.
104. Fu S, Zhang N, Yopp AC et al. TGF-beta Induces Foxp3 $^+$ T-Regulatory Cells from CD4 $^+$ CD25 - Precursors. Am J Transplant 2004; 4:1614-1627.
105. Schramm C, Huber S, Protschka M et al. TGF-beta regulates the CD4$^+$CD25$^+$ T-cell pool and the expression of Foxp3 in vivo. Int Immunol 2004; 16:1241-1249.
106. Park HB, Paik DJ, Jang E et al. Acquisition of anergic and suppressive activities in transforming growth factor-beta-costimulated CD4$^+$CD25- T cells. Int Immunol 2004; 16:1203-1213.
107. Cobbold SP, Castejon R, Adams E et al. Induction of foxP3$^+$ regulatory T cells in the periphery of T cell receptor transgenic mice tolerized to transplants. J Immunol 2004; 172:6003-6010.
108. Zheng SG, Wang JH, Gray JD et al. Natural and induced CD4$^+$CD25$^+$ cells educate CD4$^+$CD25- cells to develop suppressive activity: The role of IL-2, TGF-beta, and IL-10. J Immunol 2004; 172:5213-5221.
109. Fantini MC, Becker C, Monteleone G et al. Cutting edge: TGF-beta induces a regulatory phenotype in CD4$^+$CD25- T cells through Foxp3 induction and down-regulation of Smad7. J Immunol 2004; 172:5149-5153.
110. Flanders KC. Smad3 as a mediator of the fibrotic response. Int J Exp Pathol 2004; 85:47-64.
111. Gorelik L, Flavell RA. Transforming growth factor-beta in T-cell biology. Nat Rev Immunol 2002; 2:46-53.
112. Reed SG. TGF-beta in infections and infectious diseases. Microbes Infect 1999; 1:1313-1325.

113. Chesnoy S, Lee PY, Huang L. Intradermal injection of transforming growth factor-beta1 gene enhances wound healing in genetically diabetic mice. Pharm Res 2003; 20:345-350.
114. Racke MK, Dhib-Jalbut S, Cannella B et al. Prevention and treatment of chronic relapsing experimental allergic encephalomyelitis by transforming growth factor-beta 1. J Immunol 1991; 146:3012-3017.
115. Wallick SC, Figari IS, Morris RE et al. Immunoregulatory role of transforming growth factor beta (TGF-beta) in development of killer cells: Comparison of active and latent TGF-beta 1. J Exp Med 1990; 172:1777-1784.
116. Kuruvilla AP, Shah R, Hochwald GM et al. Protective effect of transforming growth factor beta 1 on experimental autoimmune diseases in mice. Proc Natl Acad Sci USA 1991; 88:2918-2921.
117. Raz E, Watanabe A, Baird SM et al. Systemic immunological effects of cytokine genes injected into skeletal muscle. Proc Natl Acad Sci 1993; 90:4523-4527.
118. Raz E, Duddler J, Lotz M et al. Modulation of disease activity in murine systemic lupus erythematosus by cytokine gene delivery. Lupus 1995; 4:286-292.
119. Gutierrez-Ramos JC, Andreu JL et al. Recovery from autoimmunity of MRL/lpr mice after infection with an interleukin-2/vaccinia recombinant virus. Nature 1990; 346:271-274.
120. Huggins ML, Huang FP, Xu D et al. Modulation of autoimmune disease in the MRL-lpr/lpr mouse by IL-2 and TGF-beta1 gene therapy using attenuated Salmonella typhimurium as gene carrier. Lupus 1999; 8:29-38.
121. Huggins ML, Huang FP, Xu D et al. Modulation of the autoimmune response in lupus mice by oral administration of attenuated Salmonella typhimurium expressing the IL-2 and TGF-beta genes. Ann NY Acad Sci 1997; 815:499-502.
122. van Beuningen HM, Glansbeek HL, van der Kraan PM et al. Osteoarthritis-like changes in the murine knee joint resulting from intra-articular transforming growth factor-beta injections. Osteoarthritis Cartilage 2000; 8:25-33.
123. Hagiwara E, Okubo T, Aoki I et al. IL-12-encoding plasmid has a beneficial effect on spontaneous autoimmune disease in MRL/MP-lpr/lpr mice. Cytokine 2000; 12:1035-41.
124. Khoury SJ, Sayegh MH. The roles of the new negative T cell costimulatory pathways in regulating autoimmunity. Immunity 2004; 20:529-38.
125. Carreno BM, Collins M. BTLA: A new inhibitory receptor with a B7-like ligand. Trends Immunol. 2003; 24:524-527.
126. Kitani A, Fuss IJ, Nakamura K et al. Treatment of experimental (Trinitrobenzene sulfonic acid) colitis by intranasal administration of transforming growth factor (TGF)-beta1 plasmid: TGF-beta1-mediated suppression of T helper cell type 1 response occurs by interleukin (IL)-10 induction and IL-12 receptor beta2 chain downregulation. J Exp Med 2000; 192:41-52.
127. Giladi E, Raz E, Karmeli F et al. Transforming growth factor-beta gene therapy ameliorates experimental colitis in rats. Eur J Gastroenterol Hepatol 1995; 7:341-347.
128. Song XY, Gu M, Jin WW et al. Plasmid DNA encoding transforming growth factor-beta1 suppresses chronic disease in a streptococcal cell wall-induced arthritis model. J Clin Invest 1998; 101:2615-2621.
129. Qin L, Chavin KD, Ding Y et al. Gene transfer for transplantation. Prolongation of allograft survival with transforming growth factor-beta 1. Ann Surg 1994; 220:508-518.
130. Qin L, Chavin KD, Ding Y et al. Multiple vectors effectively achieve gene transfer in a murine cardiac transplantation model. Immuno suppression with TGF-beta 1 or vIL-10. Transplantation 1995; 59:809-816.
131. Qin L, Ding Y, Bromberg JS. Gene transfer of transforming growth factor-beta 1 prolongs murine cardiac allograft survival by inhibiting cell-mediated immunity. Hum Gene Ther 1996; 7:1981-1988.
132. Chan SY, Goodman RE, Szmuszkovicz JR et al. DNA-liposome versus adenoviral mediated gene transfer of transforming growth factor beta1 in vascularized cardiac allografts: Differential sensitivity of $CD4^+$ and $CD8^+$ T cells to transforming growth factor beta1. Transplantation 2000; 70:1292-1301.
133. Hill N, Sarvetnick N. Cytokines: Promoters and dampeners of autoimmunity. Curr Opin Immunol 2002; 14:791-797.

134. Gallichan WS, Balasa B, Davies JD et al. Pancreatic IL-4 expression results in islet-reactive Th2 cells that inhibit diabetogenic lymphocytes in the nonobese diabetic mouse. J Immunol 1999; 163:1696-1703.
135. Ishii KJ, Weiss WR, Ichino M et al. Activity and safety of DNA plasmids encoding IL-4 and IFN gamma. Gene Ther 1999; 6:237-244.
136. Cameron MJ, Strathdee CA, Holmes KD et al. Biolistic-mediated interleukin 4 gene transfer prevents the onset of type 1 diabetes. Hum Gene Ther 2000; 11:1647-1656.
137. Cameron MJ, Arreaza GA, Waldhauser L et al. Immunotherapy of spontaneous type 1 diabetes in nonobese diabetic mice by systemic interleukin-4 treatment employing adenovirus vector-mediated gene transfer. Gene Ther 2000; 7:1840-1846.
138. Croxford JL, Triantaphyllapoulos K, Podhajcer LL et al. Cytokine gene therapy in experimental allergic encephalomyelitis by injection of plasmid DNA-cationic liposome complex into the central nervous system. J Immunol 1998; 160:5181-5187.
139. Moore KW, de Waal Malefyt R et al. Interleukin-10 and the interleukin-10 receptor. Annu Rev Immunol 2001; 19:683-765.
140. Weiss E, Mamelak AJ, La Morgia S et al. The role of interleukin 10 in the pathogenesis and potential treatment of skin diseases. J Am Acad Dermatol 2004; 50:657-675.
141. Groux H, Cottrez F. The complex role of interleukin-10 in autoimmunity. J Autoimmun 2003; 20:281-285.
142. Roncarolo MG, Battaglia M, Gregori S. The role of interleukin 10 in the control of autoimmunity. J Autoimmun 2003; 20:269-272.
145. Bettelli E, Nicholson LB, Kuchroo VK. IL-10, a key effector regulatory cytokine in experimental autoimmune encephalomyelitis. J Autoimmun 2003; 20:265-267.
146. Asadullah K, Sterry W, Volk HD. Interleukin-10 therapy—review of a new approach. Pharmacol Rev 2003; 55:241-269.
147. Nitta Y, Tashiro F, Tokui M et al. Systemic delivery of interleukin 10 by intramuscular injection of expression plasmid DNA prevents autoimmune diabetes in nonobese diabetic mice. Hum Gene Ther 1998; 9:1701-1707.
148. Koh JJ, Ko KS, Lee M et al. Degradable polymeric carrier for the delivery of IL-10 plasmid DNA to prevent autoimmune insulitis of NOD mice. Gene Ther 2000; 7:2099-2104.
149. Ko KS, Lee M, Koh JJ et al. Combined administration of plasmids encoding IL-4 and IL-10 prevents the development of autoimmune diabetes in nonobese diabetic mice. Mol Ther 2001; 4:313-316.
150. Lee M, Ko KS, Oh S et al. Prevention of autoimmune insulitis by delivery of a chimeric plasmid encoding interleukin-4 and interleukin-10. J Control Release 2003; 88:333-342.
151. Zhang ZL, Shen SX, Lin B et al. Intramuscular injection of interleukin-10 plasmid DNA prevented autoimmune diabetes in mice. Acta Pharmacol Sin 2003; 24:751-756.
152. Watanabe K, Nakazawa M, Fuse K et al. Protection against autoimmune myocarditis by gene transfer of interleukin-10 by electroporation. Circulation 2001; 104:1098-1100.
153. Nakano A, Matsumori A, Kawamoto S et al. Cytokine gene therapy for myocarditis by in vivo electroporation. Hum Gene Ther 2001; 12:1289-1297.
154. Adachi O, Nakano A, Sato O et al. Gene transfer of Fc-fusion cytokine by in vivo electroporation: Application to gene therapy for viral myocarditis. Gene Ther 2002; 9:577-583.
155. Zhang ZL, Lin B, Yu LY et al. Gene therapy of experimental autoimmune thyroiditis mice by in vivo administration of plasmid DNA coding for human interleukin-10. Acta Pharmacol Sin 2003; 24:885-890.
156. Batteux F, Trebeden H, Charreire J. Curative treatment of experimental autoimmune thyroiditis by in vivo administration of plasmid DNA coding for interleukin-10. Eur J Immunol 1999; 29:958-963.
157. Li MC, He SH. IL-10 and its related cytokines for treatment of inflammatory bowel disease. World J Gastroenterol 2004; 10:620-625.
158. Braat H, Peppelenbosch MP, Hommes DW. Interleukin-10-based therapy for inflammatory bowel disease. Expert Opin Biol Ther 2003; 3:725-731.
159. Prud'homme GJ. Altering immune tolerance therapeutically: The power of negative thinking. J Leukoc Biol 2004; 75:586-599.

160. Piccirillo CA, Thornton AM. Cornerstone of peripheral tolerance: Naturally occurring $CD4^+CD25^+$ regulatory T cells. Trends Immunol 2004; 25:374-380.
161. Piccirillo CA, Shevach EM. Naturally-occurring $CD4^+CD25^+$ immunoregulatory T cells: Central players in the arena of peripheral tolerance. Semin Immunol 2004; 16:81-88.
162. Sakaguchi S, Sakaguchi N, Asano M et al. Immunologic self-tolerance maintained by activated T cells expressing IL-2 receptor alpha-chains (CD25). Breakdown of a single mechanism of self-tolerance causes various autoimmune diseases. J Immunol 1995; 155:1151-1164.
163. Asano M, Toda M, Sakaguchi N et al. Autoimmune disease as a consequence of developmental abnormality of a T cell subpopulation. J Exp Med 1996; 184:387-396.
164. Sakaguchi S. Naturally arising $CD4^+$ regulatory T cells for immunologic self-tolerance and negative control of immune responses. Annu Rev Immunol 2004; 22:531-562.
165. Cottrez F, Groux H. Specialization in tolerance: Innate $CD(4^+)CD(25^+)$ versus acquired TR1 and TH3 regulatory T cells. Transplantation 2004; 77(1 Suppl):S12-5.
166. Powrie F, Read S, Mottet C et al. Control of immune pathology by regulatory T cells. Novartis Found Symp 2003; 252:92-98.
167. Peng Y, Laouar Y, Li MO et al. TGF-beta regulates in vivo expansion of Foxp3-expressing $CD4^+CD25^+$ regulatory T cells responsible for protection against diabetes. Proc Natl Acad Sci USA 2004; 101:4572-4577.
168. Santiago-Raber ML, Baccala R, Haraldsson KM et al. Type-I interferon receptor deficiency reduces lupus-like disease in NZB mice. J Exp Med 2003; 197:777-788.
169. Prud'homme GJ, Kono DH, Theofilopoulos AN. Quantitative polymerase chain reaction analysis reveals marked overexpression of interleukin-1 beta, interleukin-10 and interferon-gamma mRNA in the lymph nodes of lupus-prone mice. Mol Immunol 1995; 32:495-503.
170. Ozmen L, Roman D, Fountoulakis M et al. Experimental therapy of systemic lupus erythematosus: The treatment of NZB/W mice with mouse soluble interferon-gamma receptor inhibits the onset of glomerulonephritis. Eur J Immunol 1995; 25:6-12.
171. Kurschner C, Ozmen L, Garotta G et al. IFN-gamma receptor-Ig fusion proteins. Half-life, immunogenicity, and in vivo activity. J Immunol 1992; 149:4096-4100.
172. Kim JM, Jeong JG, Ho SH et al. Protection against collagen-induced arthritis by intramuscular gene therapy with an expression plasmid for the interleukin-1 receptor antagonist. Gene Ther 2003; 10:1543-1550.
173. Kim JM, Ho SH, Hahn W et al. Electro-gene therapy of collagen-induced arthritis by using an expression plasmid for the soluble p75 tumor necrosis factor receptor-Fc fusion protein. Gene Ther 2003; 10:1216-1224.
174. Bloquel C, Bessis N, Boissier MC et al. Gene therapy of collagen-induced arthritis by electrotransfer of human tumor necrosis factor-alpha soluble receptor I variants. Hum Gene Ther 2004; 15:189-201.
175. Gould DJ, Bright C, Chernajovsky Y. Inhibition of established collagen-induced arthritis with a tumour necrosis factor-alpha inhibitor expressed from a self-contained doxycycline regulated plasmid. Arthritis Res Ther 2004; 6:R103-113.
176. Kageyama Y, Koide Y, Uchijima M et al. Plasmid encoding interleukin-4 in the amelioration of murine collagen-induced arthritis. Arthritis Rheum 2004; 50:968-975.
177. Saidenberg-Kermanac'h N, Bessis N et al. Efficacy of interleukin-10 gene electrotransfer into skeletal muscle in mice with collagen-induced arthritis. J Gene Med 2003; 5:164-171.
178. Miyata M, Sasajima T, Sato H et al. Suppression of collagen induced arthritis in mice utilizing plasmid DNA encoding interleukin 10. J Rheumatol 2000; 27:1601-1605.
179. Campbell IL, Kay TW, Oxbrow L et al. Essential role for interferon-gamma and interleukin-6 in autoimmune insulin-dependent diabetes in NOD/WEHI mice. J Clin Invest 1991; 87:739-742.
180. Cockfield SM, Ramassar V, Urmson J et al. Multiple low dose streptozotocin induces systemic MHC expression in mice by triggering T cells to release IFN-gamma. J Immunol 1989; 142:1120-1128.
181. Sarvetnick N, Shizuru J, Liggitt D et al. Loss of pancreatic islet tolerance induced by beta-cell expression of interferon-gamma. Nature 1990; 346:844-847.
182. Matos M, Park R, Mathis D et al. Progression to islet destruction in a cyclophosphamide-induced transgenic model: A microarray overview. Diabetes 2004; 53:2310-2321.

183. Hultgren B, Huang X, Dybdal N et al. Genetic absence of gamma-interferon delays but does not prevent diabetes in NOD mice. Diabetes 1996; 45:812-817.
184. Jones SW, Souza PM, Lindsay MA. siRNA for gene silencing: a route to drug target discovery. Curr Opin Pharmacol 2004; 4:522-527.
185. Caplen NJ. Gene therapy progress and prospects. Downregulating gene expression: The impact of RNA interference. Gene Ther 2004; 11:1241-1248.
186. Ichim TE, Li M, Qian H et al. RNA interference: A potent tool for gene-specific therapeutics. Am J Transplant 2004; 4:1227-1236.
187. Wadhwa R, Kaul SC, Miyagishi M et al. Know-how of RNA interference and its applications in research and therapy. Mutat Res 2004; 567:71-84.
188. Liu J, Carmell MA, Rivas FV et al. Argonaute2 is the catalytic engine of mammalian RNAi. Science 2004; 305:1437-1441.
189. Bartel DP. MicroRNAs: Genomics, biogenesis, mechanism, and function. Cell 2004; 116:281-297.
190. Kawasaki H, Taira K. Induction of DNA methylation and gene silencing by short interfering RNAs in human cells. Nature 2004; 431:211-217.
191. McCaffrey AP, Meuse L, Pham TT et al. RNA interference in adult mice. Nature 2002; 418:38-39.
192. Lewis DL, Hagstrom JE, Loomis AG et al. Efficient delivery of siRNA for inhibition of gene expression in postnatal mice. Nat Genet 2002; 32:107-108.
193. Song E, Lee SK, Wang J et al. RNA interference targeting Fas protects mice from fulminant hepatitis. Nat Med 2003; 9:347-351.
194. Zender L, Hutker S, Liedtke C et al. Caspase 8 small interfering RNA prevents acute liver failure in mice. Proc Natl Acad Sci USA 2003; 100(13):7797-7802.
195. Hagstrom JE, Hegge J, Zhang G et al. A facile nonviral method for delivering genes and siRNAs to skeletal muscle of mammalian limbs. Mol Ther 2004; 10:386-398.
196. Kishida T, Asada H, Gojo S et al. Sequence-specific gene silencing in murine muscle induced by electroporation-mediated transfer of short interfering RNA. J Gene Med 2004; 6:105-110.
197. Devroe E, Silver PA. Therapeutic potential of retroviral RNAi vectors. Expert Opin Biol Ther 2004; 4:319-327.
198. Morris KV, Rossi JJ. Anti-HIV-1 gene expressing lentiviral vectors as an adjunctive therapy for HIV-1 infection. Curr HIV Res 2004; 2:185-191.
199. Radhakrishnan SK, Layden TJ, Gartel AL. RNA interference as a new strategy against viral hepatitis. Virology 2004; 323:173-181.
200. Manoj S, Babiuk LA, van Drunen Littel-van den Hurk S. Approaches to enhance the efficacy of DNA vaccines. Crit Rev Clin Lab Sci 2004; 41:1-39.
201. Prud'homme GJ. DNA vaccination against tumors. J Gene Med 2004; in press.
202. Isner JM. Myocardial gene therapy. Nature 2002; 415:234-239.
203. Freedman SB, Vale P, Kalka C et al. Plasma vascular endothelial growth factor (VEGF) levels after intramuscular and intramyocardial gene transfer of VEGF-1 plasmid DNA. Hum Gene Ther 2002; 13:1595-1603.
204. Moore AC, Hill AV. Progress in DNA-based heterologous prime-boost immunization strategies for malaria. Immunol Rev 2004; 199:126-143.
205. Moorthy VS, Imoukhuede EB, Keating S et al. Phase 1 evaluation of 3 highly immunogenic prime-boost regimens, including a 12-month reboosting vaccination, for malaria vaccination in Gambian men. Infect Dis 2004; 189:2213-2219.
206. Epstein JE, Charoenvit Y, Kester KE et al. Safety, tolerability, and antibody responses in humans after sequential immunization with a PfCSP DNA vaccine followed by the recombinant protein vaccine RTS,S/AS02A. Vaccine 2004; 22:1592-1603.
207. McConkey SJ, Reece WH, Moorthy VS et al. Enhanced T-cell immunogenicity of plasmid DNA vaccines boosted by recombinant modified vaccinia virus Ankara in humans. Nat Med 2003; 9:729-735.
208. Yoshida J, Mizuno M, Fujii M et al. Human gene therapy for malignant gliomas (glioblastoma multiforme and anaplastic astrocytoma) by in vivo transduction with human interferon beta gene using cationic liposomes. Hum Gene Ther 2004; 15:77-86.

Chapter 4

Targeting Antigen-Specific T Cells for Gene Therapy of Autoimmune Disease

Justin M. Johnson and Vincent K. Tuohy*

Abstract

One of the most exciting advances in the field of gene therapy in recent years is the establishment of the antigen-specific T cell as a vector for the delivery of genetically-derived treatment in vivo. In contrast with traditional applications of gene therapy, the unique versatility, specificity and memory of the T cell affords the researcher or clinician the ability to apply a broad range of tactics in the genetic treatment of disease. The T cell may be modified to deliver therapeutic products or regenerative products to sites of inflammation and tissue destruction. In addition, the T cell may be altered to modulate cellular interactions or to correct its own genetic defects to ameliorate disease. These genetic modification strategies as they relate to the treatment of autoimmune disease in experimental animal models will be the focus of this chapter, with particular emphasis on the analogs of multiple sclerosis (MS), insulin-dependent diabetes mellitus (IDDM) and rheumatoid arthritis (RA).

Introduction

Gene therapy, in its simplest form, can be represented by the replacement of a single missing or defective gene to correct a monogenic disorder. Human diseases of this nature, such as adenosine deaminase (ADA) deficiency or cystic fibrosis (CF), have been obvious and attractive targets for experimental gene therapy since the first human clinical trials began on ADA patients in 1990. In a broader sense, gene therapy can be considered not only the replacement of a defective endogenous gene, but can also incorporate the addition of foreign or modified genes to alter biological function. Thus, diseases which have multigenic, complex or unknown underlying pathologies, as most autoimmune diseases do, can also be candidates for gene therapy by exploiting endogenous biological control pathways or by creating new ones. These strategies can be categorized into four general groups: modification of target tissue; delivery of therapeutic product(s); delivery of regenerative product(s); and alteration of cellular interactions.

Although the field has met with some success, ADA remains the only human disease to date which has been effectively "cured" by gene therapy. Much of the initial enthusiasm surrounding early gene therapy experiments has led to disappointment, forcing a reevaluation of existing treatment strategies as they relate to established clinical goals. These goals of an ideal gene therapy design can be stated quite simply: delivery of the therapy should be appropriately targeted; the

*Vincent K. Tuohy—Department of Immunology, NB30, The Cleveland Clinic Foundation, Lerner Research Instititute, 9500 Euclid Avenue, Cleveland, Ohio 44195, U.S.A. Email: tuohyv@ccf.org

Gene Therapy of Autoimmune Disease, edited by Gérald J. Prud'homme. ©2005 Eurekah.com and Kluwer Academic / Plenum Publishers.

expression of the product should be long-term; and most importantly, it should be well-regulated. Any novel gene therapy scheme should be evaluated based on these three principles.

One of the most exciting and perhaps most promising strategies which has emerged in recent years is the use of antigen-specific T cells as delivery vectors for gene therapy. The T cell is an ideal vector for many reasons. First, it can accomplish all three goals of an ideal gene therapy design. The major hallmarks of immunity are specificity and memory. By nature, a T cell is uniquely suited to home to a specific antigen nearly anywhere in the body, providing exquisite targeting ability. T cells are also long-lived, thus providing potential for long-term expression of transgene(s). By incorporating an appropriate inducible promoter to drive expression of the transgene, tight regulation can be achieved. Moreover, T cells have been successfully employed in all four general gene therapy strategies either directly or indirectly. It is only in a small number of cases in which the T cell itself contains the genetic defect, as in ADA, does the T cell become the target tissue modified. The latter three categories, encompassing the delivery of therapeutic products, regenerative products and the alteration of cellular interactions provide countless possibilities for exploiting the potential of antigen-specific T cells in the treatment of autoimmune disease. These experimental applications will be the focus of this chapter.

Genetic Modification of T Cells

One misconception about the T cell is that it is extremely resistant to genetic modification. While it is true that T cells prove relatively more difficult than other types of cells, efficient DNA uptake can be achieved through a variety of techniques. A summary of these techniques appears in Table 1. All approaches fall into two broad categories: nonviral (usually plasmid) DNA uptake, termed "transfection," and viral-assisted DNA uptake, termed "transduction." Each approach has associated pros and cons. Generally, nonviral methods tend to be less efficient but very stable and with fewer side effects, while viral methods are highly efficient but come at the cost of significant drawbacks including potentially serious side effects.[1]

Viral vectors, nevertheless, dominate the field of gene therapy. All viral vectors are engineered to be replication-deficient so as to minimize risk of infection to the host. Retroviral vectors are highly effective, but are limited in that they can only transduce actively dividing cells. Interestingly, Costa et al[2] have exploited this "defect" to specifically transduce only rare populations of antigen-specific T cells which are dividing in response to cognate antigen. In contrast, adenoviral vectors have the capability of transducing both actively dividing and non-dividing cells. However, they, as well as retroviral vectors, are subject to transient gene expression, gene silencing and positional effects. They also tend to induce a strong immune response in the host, a caveat of all virally-mediated therapies. While the majority of viral gene therapy experiments have been carried out using retroviral and adenoviral vectors, vectors based on adeno-associated virus (AAV), herpes simplex virus (HSV) and cytomegalovirus (CMV) have

Table 1. Viral and nonviral methods used to genetically modify T cells

Nonviral Methods	Viral Vectors
DEAE/dextran	Retrovirus
DMSO/Polybrene	Adenovirus
Calcium phosphate co-precipitation	Adeno-associated virus (AAV)
Cationic liposome	Herpes simplex virus (HSV)
Electroporation	Cytomegalovirus (CMV)
Direct microinjection	Lentivirus
Biolistic particle ("gene gun")	

also been used. One of the most promising novel vectors is based on lentivirus. Lentiviral vectors, like adenoviral vectors, incorporate into both dividing and nondividing cells, but they are not prone to gene silencing and do not elicit a strong host immune response. In addition, being derived from HIV, they are naturally well-suited for infection of T cells. On the other hand, the fact that they are HIV-derived raises the most serious threat of all viral-based therapies: the return of replication competence. In the case of HIV, this event would obviously be catastrophic; however, even "safe" viruses such as adenovirus could wreak havoc in an immunocomprimised or seriously ill patient. Notwithstanding this possibility, there is still the risk that vector integration could cause malignant transformations of the host's tissues or cause unexpected complications related to the condition being treated. Still, viral-mediated gene transfer remains the leading technology in the field today.

Another approach which is being actively explored is the use of stem cells for gene therapy. Stem cells come in a variety of forms, but of particular interest to the immunologist is the hematopoetic stem cell (HSC). HSCs are capable of repopulating the entire hematopoetic compartment, including the immune system, thus making them perfect candidates for gene therapy strategies.[3] By targeting long-term progenitor cells with the appropriate promoter, expression of the transgene of interest can be limited to a particular lineage. Whereas plasmid DNA and viral DNA can be deployed in vivo or ex vivo, depending on the therapeutic approach, HSCs are almost exclusively modified ex vivo and returned to host to repopulate the hematopoetic system. They have proven effective as vectors in the genetic treatment of human ADA-SCID.[4]

Finally, a continuous source of genetically-modified T cells can be created by producing a transgenic animal. By microinjection of DNA into a fertilized egg, all the cells of the resulting animal can potentially express the transgene. T cells can then be harvested from that animal, or alternatively, gene expression can be limited to T cells alone via a T cell-specific promoter such as *lck* or CD4, thus allowing direct experimentation. Once established, a transgenic line becomes an invaluable tool; however, generation of a stable transgenic line is replete with pitfalls. Complications can arise from deleterious or lethal genes. The gene may not express or may not penetrate all tissues, resulting in a "mosaic" animal. The gene may fail to incorporate into the germ line, or may simply fail to transmit to offspring. Despite these limitations, transgenic animals remain an attractive tool to investigators.

In summary, these four general methods for T cell genetic modification have been applied in countless studies across a wide variety of animal models of human autoimmune disease. Practically all available autoimmune models have been studied; however, by far the most published work has been on the "big three:" experimental autoimmune encephalomyelitis (EAE), nonobese diabetic (NOD) mice and collagen-induced arthritis (CIA). These models correspond to the human diseases multiple sclerosis (MS), insulin-dependent diabetes mellitus (IDDM) and rheumatoid arthritis (RA), respectively. These models will be the primary focus for the animal studies reviewed in this chapter.

Animal Studies: Therapeutic Products

As previously stated, gene therapy may be viewed as the addition of normal, foreign or modified genes to alter biological function in order to treat a disease. The simplest application of this principle is to deliver a therapeutic product to the appropriate site. Conventional medical treatment of disease usually involves systemic administration of drugs, and this approach invariably produces unwanted side effects. In the case of autoimmune diseases, treatment protocols typically entail general immunosuppression, which can involve systemic toxicity and increased risk of infections and malignancies. An antigen-specific T cell mediated gene therapy approach can circumvent these risks by delivering a therapeutic product encoded by a gene directly to the target tissues in a controlled manner. The delivered product can be encoded by a modified or foreign gene, but more often than not, normal signaling molecules are used to exploit native biological pathways already in place. A key example of this approach is the use of immunomodulatory cytokines or their antagonists to mediate the autoimmune activity, usually toward an anti-inflammatory Th2 type response.

One of the early studies using this method involved treatment of EAE with the Th2 cytokine interleukin-4 (IL-4). EAE is a widely-studied animal model of the human disease MS.[5] As in MS, EAE pathology includes inflammatory lesions of the CNS with perivascular infiltrates. Progression of disease leads to loss of myelin accompanied by paralysis and disability. EAE can be experimentally induced by immunizing with whole proteins or synthetic peptides of myelin, such as proteolipid protein (PLP), myelin basic protein (MBP) or myelin oligodendrocyte glycoprotein (MOG). EAE can also be adoptively transferred using $CD4^+$ Th1 cells from an immunized animal. Shaw et al[6] transduced a T cell hybridoma specific for the peptide MBP 87-99 with a viral vector which constitutively expresses IL-4. The authors used a hybridoma due to their inability to transduce primary T cell lines at that time. IL-4 was chosen as the therapeutic product because it is a Th2 cytokine which inhibits Th1 induction and macrophage activation. By targeting the cells to a myelin protein, the therapy would be naturally directed to active CNS lesions. Transduced cells were injected into EAE hosts ten days after active immunization with MBP 87-99, but before first clinical signs of disease. The results showed that the treatment ameliorated the disease, and was antigen-specific in nature. However, the treatment regimen was not conducted after clinical manifestation of disease, which would have more accurately mimicked an application in human MS treatment. Moreover, no attempt was made to regulate the expression of IL-4. However, the most critical flaw was the use of hybridoma cells as the delivery vector. As these cells give rise to malignant tumors, this approach has no practical human therapeutic value. Despite these shortcomings, important proof-of-principle was established.

Similarly, our laboratory targeted EAE with the Th2 cytokine interleukin-10 (IL-10).[7] However, in contrast to the previously described study, our construct was a nonviral plasmid which we used to transfect normal T cells specific for PLP 139-151 using a DMSO/Polybrene method. Additionally, regulation was achieved using an interleukin-2 (IL-2) promoter which is normally active upon antigen engagement and is capable of driving high-level gene expression. IL-10, like IL-4, is an anti-inflammatory Th2 cytokine. Its biological functions include downregulation of MHC II expression on antigen-presenting cells (APCs), inhibition of T cell costimulatory pathways and inhibition of interferon-gamma (IFNγ) secretion by Th1 cells. These cells proved to be therapeutic when injected into EAE host mice both before and after onset of clinical symptoms, thus truly mimicking an application in human MS therapy. These cells were shown to be antigen-specific, inducible and of normal phenotype. In addition, by avoiding a viral vector, viral-associated problems were precluded.

This type of cytokine gene therapy has also been effectively demonstrated in NOD mice. The NOD mouse provides a useful model for human IDDM, also known as Type I diabetes mellitus, which is characterized by autoimmune destruction of pancreatic islet β-cells.[8] The NOD mouse spontaneously develops diabetes preceded by insulitis—an inflammation and infiltration of T cells into the islets of Langerhans. Disease can also be adoptively transferred to a susceptible host with T cells from a diabetic NOD mouse. The Th1 cytokines interleukin-1 (IL-1), tumor necrosis factor-alpha (TNFα), TNFβ, and IFNγ have all been implicated in disease pathology. Thus, strategies have surrounded either blocking the actions of these cytokines, or counteracting their effects with Th2 cytokine administration.

Moritani et al[9] generated islet-specific Th1 clones from autoreactive islet infiltrates of NOD mice and transduced these clones with a viral vector that constitutively expresses IL-10. The transduced cells were adoptively transferred into NOD mice at a 1:1 wild-type:transduced ratio. Under these conditions, a reduced incidence and severity of disease was observed in the treated animals. RT-PCR analysis showed reduced levels of IFNγ mRNA and increased levels of IL-10 mRNA in recipient islets. However, no regulatory control over the IL-10 was incorporated into the design, and the therapy was administered at the induction of disease, not after clinical onset.

Yamamoto et al[10] similarly used a viral vector to constitutively deliver IL-4 to treat diabetes in NOD mice. However, rather than targeting cells responding to a particular antigen, this study targeted T cells of a particular subtype, those bearing CD62L. The CD62L marker was chosen because it is present on $CD4^+$ regulatory cells which inhibit disease, but not present on $CD4^+$ or $CD8^+$ diabetogenic effector cells. The fact that both $CD62L^+$ and $CD62L^-$ subsets are present during all stages of disease suggests that a natural yet abortive inhibitory mechanism exists, and with facilitation, could prove therapeutic. While transduced $CD62L^-$ cells remained pathogenic, the immunoregulatory ability of $CD62L^+$ cells was greatly enhanced. In mixed cotransfer studies, the immunoregulatory cells inhibited disease induction in hosts. Although once again no attempt was made to regulate IL-4 production, nor was any post-onset therapy attempted, this study illustrates that subset targeting may improve existing gene therapy designs, and more importantly, that natural anti-autoimmune mechanisms can be enhanced and exploited to ameliorate disease.

Cytokine gene therapy has also been successfully applied in the CIA model. This model closely mimics human RA, characterized by synovitis and destruction of articular tissue. Evidence suggests that the disease is mediated by $CD4^+$ T cells.[11] Th1 cells secreting IFNγ are critical in disease development, whereas Th2 cytokines such as IL-4 or IL-10 are protective. Bessis et al[12] showed that transfected CHO fibroblasts expressing IL-4 or IL-13 can ameliorate disease. Like the EAE model, CIA can be induced either by active immunization with antigen (usually collagen type II, abbreviated CII) or by adoptive transfer of immunogenic cells from an immunized donor. Chernajovsky et al[13] transduced such immunogenic splenocytes from CII-primed mice with a viral construct designed to constitutively express transforming growth factor-beta-1 (TGFβ1). TGFβ1 exhibits multiple immunosuppressive effects and is known to correlate with recovery and/or protection in autoimmune diseases.[14] When injected into susceptible hosts, the transduced cells not only failed to confer disease, but proved to be therapeutic even when transferred into mice with established disease. Like the Moritani NOD study, antigen-targeting was provided by the native immunogenic repertoire. Likewise, no regulation of expression was attempted. Importantly, though, this study demonstrates a post-onset therapy potential, a critical prerequisite to human therapy.

Although most cytokine gene therapy designs involve direct secretion of an anti-inflammatory Th2 cytokine to inhibit disease, secretion of a Th1 cytokine antagonist can be equally as potent. A fine example of this aim is the use of interleukin-12 (IL-12) p40 dimer to block the action of the Th1 cytokine IL-12. In vivo, IL-12 exists as a heterodimer comprised of distinct subunits known as p40 and p35. Whereas the p40 subunit is responsible for the binding action of the molecule, the p35 subunit is necessary for proper signal transduction; without it, the p40 monomer or homodimer acts as an IL-12 antagonist by binding receptor without signaling. In heterodimer form, IL-12 serves as a powerful Th1 cytokine which induces IFNγ production as well as other inflammatory cytokines and may play a critical role in RA pathology; thus interference with its action provides a possible therapeutic tactic. Nakajima et al[15] transduced CII-specific T cell hybridomas as well as primary T cell lines with a viral construct encoding IL-12 p40 along with an IRES (*I*nternal *R*ibosome *E*ntry *S*ite) sequence and a luminescent reporter gene. The IRES sequence allows coexpression of two distinct genes from a single mRNA transcript. In this case, patterns of p40 expression could be visualized via the reporter gene. Transduced cells were injected during disease induction with CII immunization, but prior to first clinical signs. Disease was clearly ameliorated and only CII-specific cells had a therapeutic effect. Additionally, the homing behavior of the transferred cells to affected joints was demonstrated using real-time bioluminescent imaging.

However, again no regulatory control over expression was imposed, the therapy was begun prior to onset of disease, and although transduced primary T cells were effective in treating the disease, they were markedly less effective than the transduced hybridomas, whose tumorigenic properties render them unusable as vectors for human therapy. This study does however illustrate the potential for evaluating antigen-specific therapies by using imaging techniques to elucidate local delivery patterns in vivo.

On a final note, antigen-specific T cell delivery of therapeutic products may not necessarily be restricted to traditional autoimmune diseases; this type of strategy has also been examined in transplant rejection models. While autoimmune diseases can be distilled into a "self" versus "nonself" paradigm, a transplanted organ physiologically becomes part of the "self," and thus immune rejection may in a sense constitute autoimmunity. A longstanding goal of transplantation is to manipulate T cells to accept the foreign tissue as "self." To date, this remains a daunting task. However, a clever study by Hammer et al[16] takes advantage of the natural tendency for T cells to home and migrate into allografts to potentially deliver therapeutic product(s) to minimize rejection. In this study, allo-specific T cells were transduced ex vivo with a viral construct constitutively expressing enhanced green fluorescent protein (EGFP) and transferred back into host rats with various graft types. The EGFP reporter was detected at high levels in the transplants of rats with allografts, but not in syngeneic or third-party grafts. This demonstrated the efficacy and antigen-specificity of the design. While no actual therapeutic payload was delivered, proof-of-principle of this approach was established.

Animal Studies: Regenerative Products

Regenerative product delivery is a natural extension and progression from therapeutic product delivery. The obvious first step in combating an autoimmune disease is to stop the immune onslaught. However, this may not necessarily represent a "cure." Because tissue destruction is frequently involved in disease pathology, tissue regeneration may be necessary to exact a complete recovery. This may include repair of damaged tissue, generation of new or artificial tissue, or both. In light of recent studies, it has become clear that during autoimmunity self-suppression and/or tissue regeneration to some degree does occur. Affected organs are not merely passive targets of autoimmune disease, but actively resist using endogenous systems.[14] If autoimmune disease is a failure of these natural systems to completely harness self-reactivity and repair damaged tissues, then obviously restoring or facilitating these abilities would provide an incredibly powerful tool for clinical treatment. Surprisingly, though, much of the research in the field has focused only on halting the autoimmune process, with little attention given to regeneration. In RA it is virtually unexplored. In IDDM, focus is mostly on creation of de novo non-β-cell insulin secretion. Only in CNS disorders has much experimental progress been made, probably due to the immense importance of the tissue and its relative inability to heal itself.

When considering regenerative therapy of the CNS, several outmoded dogmas must be discarded. Firstly, CNS tissues do possess an innate albeit weak ability to heal. This ability can be greatly augmented by the introduction of native neural growth factors via gene therapy. Grill et al showed that fibroblasts engineered to secrete nerve growth factor (NGF) caused axon regrowth not only in acute, but in chronic CNS injury.[17] Secondly, the CNS has long been regarded an system of "immune privilege;" that immune cells are naturally excluded from entering the CNS where evolution has determined that they would do more harm than good. While the blood-brain barrier (BBB) does ordinarily hold the immune system at bay, T cells and macrophages can and do cross it during infection and injury,[18] and Schwartz et al have shown that the native immune response following CNS injury can actually be beneficial.[19] Therefore, a T cell-mediated gene therapy should be both possible and advantageous. Flügel et al have shown proof-of-principle of this approach by using T cells to deliver NGF to the CNS.[20] Thirdly, while it has long been known that MS/EAE pathology involves damage to the myelin sheath surrounding the axon,[21] only in recent years has it been show that the axon itself is also a target and consequently suffers severe damage.[22] In support of the view that intrinsic but abortive repair systems in the CNS actively participate, Mathisen et al showed evidence of autologous partial remyelination in EAE animals which directly corresponded to recovery from disease.[23] Therefore, in MS/EAE applications, products which aim to regenerate myelin and/or axons have been logical choices for investigators.

Our laboratory chose platelet-derived growth factor-A (PDGF-A) as the regenerative effector to genetically treat EAE.[24] PDGF-A is important in the development of the oligodendrocyte—the myelinating cell of the CNS and primary target in EAE and MS. PDGF-A stimulates the proliferation, migration, differentiation and survival of oligodendrocyte precursors. Our construct, like our previous IL-10 delivery vector, was a nonviral plasmid which incorporated the antigen-inducible IL-2 promoter to regulate expression of the transgene. And similar to the prior study, normal T cells targeted to the myelin epitope PLP 139-151 were transfected using a DMSO/Polybrene method. Cells were fluorescently labeled with PKH26 for tracking purposes and injected into actively immunized EAE mice three days after clinical onset of disease. Bioassays revealed studies that the transfected T cells did indeed produce biologically active PDGF-A and cell tracking showed that they in fact migrated to the CNS. Ongoing disease was significantly ameliorated, demonstrating a true therapeutic effect. Not only does this study illustrate an effective treatment strategy for degenerative CNS diseases, but it also shows proof-of-principle that T cells are capable of expressing fully active "nonclassical" cytokines.

While regenerative therapy may be applied secondarily to halting the autoimmune process, the two aims could potentially be overlapped to provide a synergistic therapy. In fact, the two may even be one in the same. One such case exists in the actions of NGF. In the CNS, NGF plays a pivotal role in the survival and differentiation of select neuronal populations. In addition, it exhibits immunomodulatory effects such as suppression of MHC II inducibilty in microglia and stimulation of memory B cells and Th2 responses. Flügel et al[20] tested NGF gene therapy in the EAE model. In that study, MBP-specific T cell lines were transduced with a viral construct encoding NGF. These cells were adoptively transferred alone or cotransferred with wild-type MBP-specific immunogenic T cells. The transduced cells alone were incapable of causing disease, and more importantly, suppressed disease in cotransfer experiments. Histological examination of the CNS revealed that the therapy also decreased infiltration of inflammatory cells. This property was also confirmed with an in vitro BBB model. These data suggested that NGF, acting through its receptor, p75, hindered the ability of monocytes/macrophages to cross the BBB, thus providing a therapeutic effect. While this study made no attempt at regulation of expression and inhibited induction of EAE rather than treating ongoing disease, it demonstrated the potential of both NGF and the targeting of the BBB in autoimmune CNS therapy. Disappointingly, though, the authors made no attempt to explore the regenerative possibilities of the therapy.

Animal Studies: Alteration of Cellular Interactions

Of the four general categories of T cell gene therapy, this one is by far the most diverse, and exists because these studies do not conform nicely into previous categories, yet they may encompass elements of one or more simultaneously. In a generic sense, delivery of a cytokine may itself be considered an alteration of cellular interactions; however for this discussion we will primarily be concerned with genetic manipulations of intercellular functions such as: modulation of signaling pathways; apoptosis induction; "vetoing;" inhibition of epitope spreading; tolerance induction; tolerance reversal; and specificity programming.

One study in which an attempt was made to interrupt a Th1 signaling pathway was conducted by Chen et al in the CIA model.[25] In this study, a CIA-susceptible transgenic mouse line expressing a hybrid IL-2/IL-4 receptor on its T cells was generated. In response to IL-2 secretion, which normally occurs in the T cell upon antigen engagement, the receptor transduces a Th2-type IL-4 signal instead of its native Th1-type IL-2 signal. Other than this type-2 response to antigen engagement, the T cells were phenotypically normal. Since Th2 responses are generally regarded as beneficial in autoimmune diseases, including RA/CIA, it was hypothesized that these animals would be protected from disease upon priming with CII. Surprisingly, the converse turned out to be true; the disease was greatly exacerbated with a greater incidence, accelerated onset and increased severity versus controls. Although the antigen-specific proliferation of these transgenic cells was normal, and their cytokine profiles were typical of the anticipated Th2 phenotype, histological examination of the arthritic joints revealed a substantial recruitment of eosinophils. Because eosinophils are capable of tissue damage and the recruitment of additional inflammatory cells, they may represent a local pathological mediator. This finding suggests that a Th2-type response may play a role in disease pathogenesis, at least in this model, and raises an important caveat for all Th2-based therapies. This interpretation has been supported by a number of other recent studies which show Th2 pathogenesis in EAE and NOD models.[26,27]

Another strategy for curtailing the propagation of potentially harmful inflammatory events lies in the blockade of T cell costimulatory signals. In order to become activated, a T cell not only needs to have presentation of antigen via MHC to its T cell receptor (TCR) in the context of an antigen-presenting cell (APC), but also requires a second signal mediated through the additional binding of receptors and ligands between these two cells. In the absence of this second signal, T cells will undergo anergy or apoptosis. This system is believed to be a natural failsafe mechanism to discourage naïve T cells from responding to self. As such, it provides a logical basis for an exogenous therapy. The T cell surface receptors CD28 and CD40L and their respective APC binding partners B7/CTLA4 and CD40 have been shown to be important in costimulation. Matsui et al targeted these molecules with antagonists delivered by adenoviral vectors.[28] These vectors produce IgG fusion proteins of either CTLA4 or CD40, which inhibit binding of the native ligands. The model system tested was experimental autoimmune myocarditis (EAM), an analog of human myocarditis which is induced in animals by immunization with cardiac myosin. Intravenous injections of the vector(s) were administered either at induction of disease with the priming antigen or two weeks later, following clinical onset. Treatment at induction completely inhibited disease, and treatment post-onset was also remarkably effective. This represents an important finding, for it suggests a relevant clinical application in human myocarditis.

A strategically different approach to halting the autoimmune response relies not merely on downregulation of the responding cells, but seeks to actively kill them. One method of accomplishing this is to exploit the natural pathways of apoptosis, or programmed cell death. Apoptosis can be triggered by means of the Fas receptor and Fas ligand (FasL) circuit. Upon engagement of Fas, FasL induces a death signal in the target cell. This mechanism is necessary in many biological systems to sustain normal function, and is believed to play an important role in maintaining self-tolerance. Fas is expressed constitutively on most tissues and is normally upregulated during inflammation, including on the activated synovial cells and infiltrating leukocytes responsible for the pathology of CIA/RA. Despite this inherent upregulation of Fas, FasL expression in the inflamed joint remains low. Zhang et al hypothesized that upregulation of FasL at the arthritic site would counteract the massive infiltration of inflammatory cells which mediate the disease and would thus reverse its course.[29] This group devised an adenoviral vector which constitutively expresses FasL and injected it directly into the joints of mice with CII-induced CIA three days after onset of disease. This therapy proved effective in ameliorating the ongoing disease. The beneficial effect was directly attributed to FasL, as the effect was nullified when a Fas-blocking agent was introduced. However, as the authors point out, the adenoviral vector was relatively short-lived due to its clearance by the host's immune system. This would obviate the need to incorporate any sort of regulatory mechanism into the vector design, although an effective clinical therapy regimen would involve multiple intra-articular injections over time. This would, however, be preferable to direct injections of even shorter-lived nongenetically-derived therapeutic agents into the joints.

An additional method for the direct elimination of disease-mediating cells builds upon yet another intrinsic mechanism for harnessing self-reactivity. It has been proposed that a natural mechanism exists in which one $CD8^+$ T cell may present a self-peptide/MHC complex to an autoreactive $CD8^+$ T cell and eliminate or regulate it. This process has been described as "vetoing." Thus, the creation of a veto-like cell through genetic modification could prove therapeutic in autoimmune disease. This type of targeting of the autoimmune effector cell is precisely what was performed in an elegant EAE study by Jyothi et al.[30] This study was conducted using a transgenic mouse that expresses a chimeric receptor on all its T cells. The hybrid receptor consists of an MHC II molecule complexed with a self-epitope of the CNS, MBP 89-101. The MHC is subsequently linked to the cytoplasmic activation domains of TCR. Thus, engagement of this cell with a TCR specific for its "bait," the self-peptide, activates it. The type of activation that results depends on the phenotype of the cell possessing the chimeric receptor. For the purposes of this study, the transgenic cells were differentiated into cytotoxic lymphocytes (CTLs) thus enabling cytotoxic destruction of the target autoreactive population. These cells were transferred into hosts primed for EAE with MBP 89-101 either at the time of immunization or after onset of clinical disease. In both cases, the transferred cells greatly reduced disease severity. Even after the specificity of the autoimmune repertoire had "spread" to additional myelin self-epitopes, these neo-autoreactive cells were also suppressed. This may be due to the fact that the treatment also caused a Th2 phenotype shift in the remaining MBP-specific cells, either by guiding the development or expansion of the Th2 cells, or by selectively killing only Th1-type responders. In any case, this Th2 shift, which was evidenced by increased IL-4 production, may have afforded additional protection from disease beyond the targeted destruction of the Th1-type priming repertoire. As this approach proved effective in treating ongoing disease, this study illustrates a novel method of targeting autoimmunity that has great potential clinical relevance. Because it can be adapted to a variety of situations by altering the effector cell type, antigen and signal transduced, this technique may yield even further applications.

The concept of epitope spreading, briefly alluded to in the previous study, warrants a thorough discussion as it has great implications for all antigen-specific therapies, and can itself be targeted for arresting autoimmune disease. Epitope spreading can be defined as acquired neo-autoreactivity to epitopes not initially involved in disease. This can be attributed to the endogenous self-priming that occurs when previously sequestered self-epitopes enter the inflammatory milieu as a result of tissue breakdown. This phenomenon has been demonstrated in EAE and MS and may provide an underlying mechanism for the relapses and remissions exhibited in both.[31] As the response to the initial epitope wanes during remission, response to a new self-epitope may be acquired resulting in relapse. The pattern of epitope recognition during EAE in the SWXJ mouse when primed with PLP 139-151 exhibits a predictable and invariable sequence: PLP 139-151 → PLP 249-273 → MBP 87-99 → PLP 173-198.[32] The fact that this sequence of acquired self-reactivity is predicable suggests that clinical intervention in this cascade may provide a basis for therapy. Our laboratory explored this possibility by injecting the previously described genetically-engineered T cells that secrete IL-10 in response to antigen engagement.[33] However in this case, the cells generated were specific for the antigen MBP 87-99, which is a spreading epitope identified in the predictable cascade, rather than the priming antigen, PLP 139-151. Treatment was initiated two days after onset of clinical symptoms. As predicted, these cells dramatically ameliorated disease, while transfected T cells specific for a nonself antigen or a nonspreading myelin epitope did not. Moreover, it was observed that the source of IL-10 eventually shifted from the transferred cells to the native T cell population, suggesting that transferred cells had induced host-derived protection. Although this study provides proof-of-principle that preemptive targeting of the epitope spreading cascade in established disease is therapeutic, deployment of this type of therapy in human MS may prove challenging. Firstly, the priming event cannot be predicted and the priming antigen is not known. Secondly, whereas a predictable cascade can be elucidated in a genetically pure mouse strain, this is not the case in the genetically diverse human population. It is not clear whether this hurdle can be overcome in order to translate this technique into human therapy. In any case, the pathologic process of epitope spreading presents an immunologic moving target that may complicate antigen-specific therapies; therefore any such proposed treatment must address this issue.

Another important native immunological system which can be advantageously manipulated through gene therapy is that of tolerance. Tolerance, simply stated, is failure to respond to an antigen. Tolerance to self is critical in maintaining normal function; if tolerance to self-antigens is lost, devastating autoimmune disease can result. Restoration of this pathologic loss of self-tolerance has long been a goal of immunology. Conventional approaches include such means as oral tolerance, wherein the patient is literally "fed" the antigen, or altered peptide ligands, modified versions of the antigen designed to coax the immune system back to a nonreactive state. While these and other conventional attempts at tolerance have revealed much about the immune system, none has proven worthy as a treatment for human autoimmune disease. Gene therapy provides a novel and hopeful strategy for bringing about this aim. One of the simplest yet paradoxically least understood ways to induce genetic tolerance is through the use of DNA vaccination. A DNA vaccine consists simply of a naked plasmid which carries the cDNA encoding the protein of choice.[34] When transferred into a host, usually by intramuscular injection, one of three outcomes is possible: the plasmid can be processed by host cells to merely produce the intended protein; the protein can further be presented to the immune system to induce anergy, or a tolerant state; or presentation could result in activation of the immune system, hence the term "vaccination." The wide variety of potential outcomes presents a puzzle but seems to depend largely on the plasmid vector and whether or not it contains immunogenic bacterial CpG motifs which generally result in activation. Despite much research in this area, the mechanism of DNA vaccination has yet to be fully elucidated. Notwithstanding, many experiments applying this strategy to autoimmune disease models have been conducted. This has led to even greater confusion, since conflicting reports have been published treating the same disease using plasmids expressing the same antigen. For example, Ruiz et al[35] showed EAE amelioration while Tsunoda et al[36] showed enhanced EAE. Both groups vaccinated with the PLP 139-151 determinant. It is obvious that more study is necessary before any human therapies are considered.

A further and perhaps more predictable method for genetic tolerance induction targets the APC. Chen et al[37] transduced B cells in such a way as to produce antigen-specific tolerance. This group constructed a retroviral vector expressing PLP 100-154 fused to a lysosomal targeting sequence to ensure proper association with MHC II. These B cells, when injected into naïve hosts, present this self-antigen to T cells in the absence of costimulatory molecules. As discussed earlier, this second signal is necessary for activation and without it T cells enter apoptosis or anergy, thus effectively tolerized. One to two weeks following transfer, mice were challenged with PLP 139-151, an immunogenic peptide traversed by construct. The tolerized mice fared better clinically than controls; the majority were protected from disease induction. Subsequent assays revealed antigen-specific T cell nonreactivity and decreased IL-2 production. However, this treatment regimen failed to protect a substantial portion of mice, and it while it may have proven preventative, post-onset therapy was not attempted.

Agarwal et al[38] conducted a similar study in the experimental autoimmune uveitis model (EAU) using an IgG-coupled antigen. EAU is an experimental model for the human retinal disease uveitis that is induced with interphotoreceptor retinoid-binding protein (IRBP). In this study, IRBP was fused to the heavy chain of IgG_1 because it has tolerogenic properties known to result in long-term suppression of the antigen-specific immune response. Like the Chen study, transduced B cells were transferred to naïve hosts, and immunization with the priming antigen occurred 10 days later. Likewise, these mice fared much better than controls in disease outcome. However in this case, post-immunization therapy was also attempted. Treatment begun seven days following priming also resulted in disease amelioration, although a much more intense regimen was required. While encouraging, it is not clear whether this type of approach would be effective in human patients with established or chronic disease, especially in light of epitope spreading. An effective clinical application would have to include every possible epitope of every possible protein target involved in that disease. Moreover, while evidence suggests that B cells are long-lived, only short-term effects were examined in these studies. Due to the problems inherent with viral vectors, the benefits noted may in fact be ephemeral.

Although it may seem counterintuitive, *reversal* of tolerance may also be beneficial in combating autoimmunity. In this case, by breaking tolerance to an inflammatory mediator such as a Th1 cytokine, the host mounts an immune response against a critical link in an ongoing autoimmune condition. The result: autoimmunity versus autoimmunity. There is some evidence to suggest that this process occurs naturally as one of the many intrinsic countermeasures against autoimmunity. And like so many other native mechanisms, gene therapy may enhance or reinstate an inadequate natural response. Wildbaum et al took advantage of this opportunity by targeting TNFα for tolerance reversal in the adjuvant-induced arthritis (AA) model.[39] AA is an alternative to the CIA model of human RA that is induced with an injection of complete Freund's adjuvant (CFA). TNFα was chosen as the target because of its potent inflammatory effects and its implication in autoimmune pathologies, particularly in RA and MS. In this study DNA vaccination was performed using a plasmid encoding TNFα and containing the immunogenic CpG motif. Disease was induced with CFA before or after DNA vaccination, and in both cases the treatment was remarkably effective. In addition, anti-TNFα antibodies were produced that surprisingly appeared to "respond" appropriately in their production, reflecting the disease state. This suggests an enhancement of a native, controlled anti-autoimmune response. Most importantly however, this study represents the critical minority of approaches in which a significant amelioration of ongoing disease was achieved. This mode of anti-TNFα therapy has also been proven effective in the EAE model.[40] Wildbaum et al also used this approach to effectively modulate a therapeutic Th1 → Th2 shift.[41] By targeting IFNγ-inducible protein-10 (IP-10), a chemokine which drives naïve T cells to a Th1 phenotype, they were able to break tolerance and induce an anti-IP-10 response in the hosts. This in turn mediated a Th2 phenotype shift which prevented EAE induction and ameliorated ongoing EAE.

As we have seen, there is an enormous array of approaches which may be undertaken in harnessing the power of the T cell to counter autoimmune disease. One final adjunct to these studies involves the genetic modification of the most essential T cell function—specificity. This inherent characteristic is what makes antigen-specific T cell therapy so attractive. It is in fact what gives a T cell its identity. And yet this quality is determined solely by the two chains of the TCR, alpha and beta. Kessels et al sought to introduce a genetically engineered TCR to T cells in order to exogenously "lock in" the target.[42] In this study, the genes encoding both chains of a TCR specific for an antigen shared by a particular tumor and influenza strain were inserted into a retroviral vector. Mouse splenocytes were transduced with the construct ex vivo and reinfused into donors. After two days, mice were challenged with the cognate influenza strain or control strain. The mice exhibited fully antigen-specific responses to the virus in vivo. The transduced T cells also proliferated normally then subsided appropriately following viral clearance. Moreover, this therapy was also effective against established tumors bearing the target antigen. Side effects, including autoimmune, were minimal. However, the viral-based treatment itself is vulnerable to immune attack; and since TCR heterodimers of endogenous/exogenous origin are possible, unpredictable and potentially harmful effects could result. Despite these concerns, this study illustrates a novel tactic with immense potential. Although designed primarily as a method to rapidly counter infections or tumors, it could certainly be deployed in antigen-specific autoimmune therapies. For instance, designer TCRs could be used in conjunction with therapeutic payloads to direct genetically-modified T cells to their appropriate targets. This example illustrates one of a myriad of ways that practically any of the approaches discussed in this chapter may be combined in a synergistic fashion.

Future Directions

It is clear from the current state of research in the field of gene therapy that great progress has been made; however in order to advance this science one must take stock of the innumerable near-misses and failures. These will no doubt aid in the design of the next generation of gene therapies which may ultimately hold the key to reversing human autoimmune disease. Several critical points should be noted when devising new strategies. Firstly, the therapy must prove effective in treating ongoing disease. A therapy which is only effective in preventing induction of an autoimmune disease is of little clinical value. Secondly, the possible deleterious effects of the therapeutic payload must be considered. The systemic, pleiotropic, long-term and unknown effects of any agent or biological manipulation need to be evaluated. While a particular therapeutic agent itself may not present any danger, simply by altering homeostatic balance other harmful effects may indirectly result. The delivery vector may also complicate the effects of the therapy; Croxford et al showed conflicting therapeutic outcomes of IL-10 in EAE when delivered via different vectors and modes.[43] Additionally, when cellular delivery vectors are used, cell type is influential. Morita et al showed disease regression in CIA when dendritic cells (DCs) were transfected, but no effect was observed when T cells or fibroblasts were used.[44] Thirdly, the delivery vector or process itself may be directly harmful to the host. Infectious viral vectors or transformation of host tissue are genuine dangers. Moreover, since so many vectors are designed with no regulatory elements in mind, one must ask if constitutive delivery of any agent is prudent. It can be assumed that it would not be beneficial to have continuous therapy after the disease or harmful condition were ameliorated. Lastly, the therapy must be designed to account for the dynamic processes of disease. These include epitope spreading, relapsing/remitting, autologous anti-autoimmune responses and other transient processes inherent in the disease course.

Current gene therapy strategies may be improved upon by the lessons learned from prior studies. First of all, better regulation and delivery of products can be achieved. Constitutive promoters may be replaced with inducible and/or tissue-specific ones. Viral delivery vectors may also be enhanced. One such recent advance is the self-inactivating (SIN) vector. A commonly observed problem associated with traditional viral vectors is that of "promoter interference," a condition which occurs when a regulatory promoter is inserted between the viral LTR promoter elements causing hindrance of one promoter or the other. This typically manifests as low gene expression with high viral titers, or vice versa. SIN vectors overcome this problem by neutralizing the 3' LTR after integration, leaving only the regulatory promoter active. Retroviral SIN vectors are commercially available[45] and lentiviral versions are currently being developed.[3] While SIN vectors offer a great advantage over traditional viral vectors, still greater efficiencies have been reported using hybrid vectors. Zhao-Emonet et al[46] eliminated the 3' LTR element altogether and replaced it with a CD4 minimal promoter/enhancer. Thus, this construct allows T cell-specific gene expression while maintaining high viral titers.

Furthermore, to improve regulation of gene expression an added level of control can be imposed on the delivery vector. Several commercially available systems allow gene expression to be turned on or off in vivo simply with the addition of an exogenous substance, such as doxycyline or rapamycin, which can be injected or simply added to the diet. The *cre/lox* system offers even greater flexibility, as the *cre* recombinase which triggers the reaction can either be added exogenously or transcribed from another vector (or even from the *same* vector) under the appropriate regulatory control. The *cre* recombinase reacts with a pair of specific target sites, termed "*lox*P," splicing out the intervening sequence. The result can be gene activation, inactivation, or a combination of both as one gene is interrupted while another is simultaneously rejoined.[47] With careful design genes can even be made to self-splice.[48] This event can be temporally and spatially controlled via appropriate promoter selection, allowing such a feat as normal development of a *cre/lox* transgenic animal before splicing occurs. While this system offers tremendous flexibility, unlike the aforementioned systems the effects are irreversible. Although this is generally considered a drawback, permanence in some designs may be desirable.

Another level of control which may be imposed is the "suicide gene," a genetic kill switch which can terminate runaway therapies or those which have simply run their course. One of the most commonly used is the herpes simplex virus thymidine kinase (HSV-TK) gene. Under normal circumstances it is harmless, but upon administration of ganciclovir it kills dividing host cells from within.[49] This technique has been used experimentally and clinically to arrest the graft-versus-host disease (GVHD) that sometimes occurs following an allogenic bone marrow graft.[50,51] Its potential in killing alloreactive T cells in early post-transplant has also been shown.[52]

Finally, current therapy systems may be improved upon by enhancing expression of the delivered product(s). The addition of a reporter gene, either alone or in tandem with an effector gene via an IRES sequence, can allow spatial and temporal evaluation of expression patterns in vivo.[3,15] Intron sequences can be incorporated into the design to enhance gene expression, and the addition of insulator elements can greatly reduce the effects of gene silencing.

While familiar strategies continue to improve, new strategies will undoubtedly emerge. New knowledge will breed new therapies. Better understanding of disease mechanisms and pathologies, along with better understanding of the mechanisms and functions of biological agents will certainly lead researchers down new paths. One historical example of this is a clinical study of MS conducted in 1987 in which patients were treated with injections of IFNγ.[53] Seven of the eighteen participants suffered severe relapses; the study was immediately halted. While it may seem counterintuitive to use an inflammatory Th1 cytokine to treat an autoimmune disease, the contemporary belief was that the pathology of MS involved an IFNγ deficiency. Additionally the disease was widely viewed as viral in nature; IFNγ also exhibits strong anti-viral properties. Its cousins, IFNα and IFNβ had already been shown to be therapeutic in MS. Therefore, based on the information available at the time, IFNγ was a rational choice. Only in retrospect does it seem otherwise, and in a similar fashion some of the therapies chosen today may seem irrational when looking back. While so many anti-autoimmune therapies are based upon Th2 mediators, one must ask if this type of cytokine skewing is prudent. The Th2 phenotype is pathological in allergy and also in the autoimmune disease systemic lupus erythematosis (SLE). It may also play a role in the pathologies of diseases classically attributed to Th1 such as CIA/RA.[25] In addition, native biologic countermeasures or redundant pathways may eventually compensate an artificial cytokine shift, thus negating the effect. In any case, future research will illuminate mistakes of the past and present and allow more appropriate choices of therapeutic agents.

New delivery vectors will also undoubtedly come into play. Science has harnessed the power of infectious viruses and rendered them replication-deficient, self-inactivating workhorses that do our bidding. We've even made an ally of HIV. What's next? The next generation of delivery vehicles may not be viral vectors or plasmids. Currently, human artificial chromosomes are

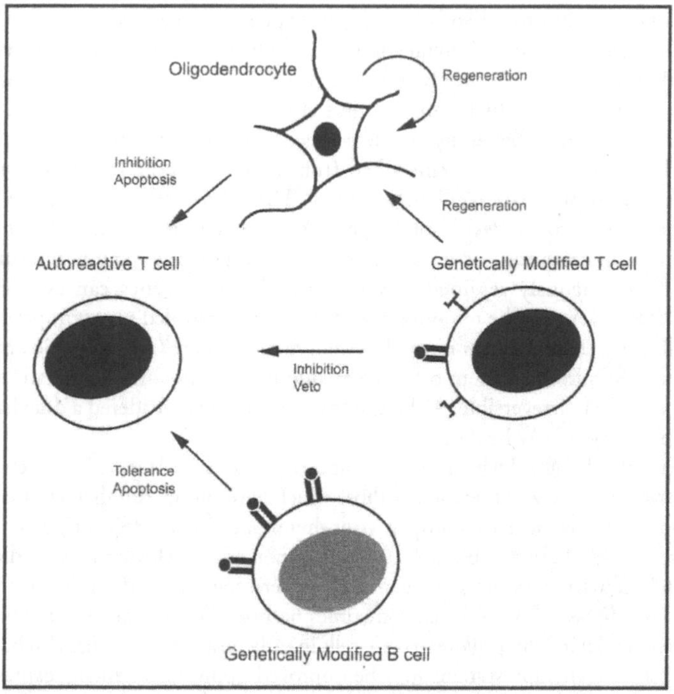

Figure 1. A schematic depiction of a hypothetical multi-pronged T cell gene therapy design. In this representative autoimmune attack on the CNS, the target tissue (the oligodendrocyte, top) has been genetically modified to resist the autoreactive T cell (left) by secreting inhibitory Th2 cytokines and inducing apoptosis of invading cells via FasL. Concurrently, the target tissue produces regenerative products to aid recovery. The genetically modified therapeutic T cell (right) inhibits the autoreactive T cell by secreting anti-inflammatory cytokines upon engagement of antigen. The antigen specificity has been encoded with custom TCRs (outer arms) and the cell also performs a "veto" function by presenting self-antigen on a chimeric MHC molecule (middle arm). Moreover, the genetically modified B cell (bottom) expresses exogenously coded self-antigen on native MHC molecules to tolerize the autoreactive cell. These multiple processes may act synergistically to inhibit disease and encourage regeneration of damaged tissue.

being developed which are capable of expressing large genes in a stable, long-term and regulated manner with a complete absence of side effects.[54] These have the distinct advantage of being a completely natural and maintainable structure in human cells. To date, proof-of-principle gene replacement therapy has been shown in vitro, but has not been tested in humans. There are many chromosomal elements that are not fully understood, particularly the centromere, which may require additional research. Furthermore, since synthetic chromosomes typically occupy several megabases of DNA, a formidable system is required for in vivo delivery.

Another possibility for gene delivery in vivo lies in gene activated matrices (GAMs). This technology consists of a matrix of solid material which can serve as a platform for the direct delivery of plasmid or viral DNA at the appropriate site.[55] Genes expressed could, for example, mediate tissue repair while the matrix serves as a scaffold for new cells. This method could be applied to autoimmune diseases with a single focus, such as IDDM, or may be applied in other ways to diseases with multiple foci. For example, one strategy might involve treatment of MS by creating a synthetic GAM "thymus" which would clonally delete self-reactive cells with FasL.

This example again invokes the potential power of combination therapies. A hypothetical multi-angled therapy approach is illustrated in Figure 1. As previously mentioned, multiple gene therapies may be combined to create a synergistic effect. Coexpression of multiple therapeutic products may exhibit this. Ko et al showed synergy in suppressing diabetes in NOD mice with coadministration of IL-4 and IL-10 in dual vectors.[56] Vectors could potentially coexpress immunomodulatory and regenerative products (or products which elicit both effects) to shut down the autoimmune response and promote healing. In a parallel therapy, target tissue may be genetically modified to induce immunoregulation, regeneration and/or apoptosis of invading immune cells. Although perhaps many years away, a novel strategy might involve transducing T cells ex vivo with a library of vectors encoding antigen-specific TCRs recognizing all potential target-tissue epitopes while coexpressing therapeutic proteins in an antigen-inducible manner. Alternately or in addition, vector libraries encoding all potential self-epitopes of target tissue may be delivered to B cells to tolerize the patient against future attacks. These strategies may also benefit from combination with traditional nongenetic medicine. This type of holistic approach may ultimately provide the maximum benefit.

Finally, the nature of autoimmunity itself is continually questioned yielding better and more useful philosophies while outmoded dogmas wither. Even the "self" versus "nonself" paradigm, a cornerstone of immunology for many decades, has been challenged. Matzinger has proposed it be replaced with a "danger" hypothesis, which purports that the immune system disregards what is self or nonself and merely responds appropriately to that which poses a threat to the body.[57] Similarly, the Th1/Th2 paradigm has been challenged. Many reports have surfaced of nonTh2 cells which appear to regulate Th1 cells. These include Tr1, Th3, natural killer (NK) T cells and autoimmune related regulatory T cells (ART).[58] Furthermore, autoimmunity is increasingly being viewed as a potentially beneficial process. Autoimmunity occurs as an innate and propitious mechanism in healthy individuals, performing critical functions such as eliminating senescent red blood cells from the body. It can play an advantageous role in CNS injury[19] and may participate in the native counter-response to harmful autoimmunity.[40] It has recently been demonstrated that adoptive induction of autoimmunity directed against melanocyte self-antigens resulted in sustained regression of metastatic melanomas in human patients.[59] While these patients subsequently suffered significant destruction of melanocytes, this type of exogenously-induced autoimmunity may provide a useful therapy for tissue-specific tumors of organs or tissues not essential for survival.

Conclusions

The preceding studies illustrate in animal models that antigen-specific T cells may indeed be effective when engaged either directly or indirectly in the treatment of human autoimmune diseases and perhaps in diseases of other modalities as well. T cells have capably met our three established goals of gene therapy, exhibiting precise targeting, long-term expression, and strict regulation of therapy delivery. They have been deployed successfully in animal models using the four general strategies outlined, delivering therapeutic products and regenerative products, participating in auspicious cellular interactions, and have themselves had genetic defects repaired to reverse disease pathology.[60] By exploiting their innate homing ability, antigen-specific T cells can be rendered "guided missiles" capable of delivering virtually any payload in a regulated manner to practically any target. While it is tempting to strive to duplicate in human clinical trials the successes apparent in animal studies, caution must be exercised. The adverse side effects associated with the therapy, including its route, delivery mode and genetic product must be considered. Long-term effects must also be evaluated, and curtailment potential should be engineered into the design. Proper correlation between animal models and human diseases should be determined, as these models do not mimic their human counterparts in every circumstance. Likewise, the human population is not homogeneic as experimental mouse strains are. Thorough understandings of human diseases and their pathologies must be achieved in order to predict and prevent negative outcomes. Lastly, ethical consideration must be given to any proposed human gene therapy.[61] Could the therapy do more harm than good? Could it be fatal? What would the impact on future generations be if the germ line were altered? These are some of the many important questions which must be addressed before human gene therapy moves into the mainstream of clinical medicine.

Although the treatment of human monogenic disorders with gene therapy is now a reality, complex autoimmune disorders will not be as easily conquered. However, the emerging view of the T cell as a tool for the therapy of autoimmune and other diseases will no doubt lead to effective clinical therapies with the potential to cure grave and devastating illnesses. It may be well into the distant future that an "off-the-shelf" genetic remedy is available for the treatment of patients; that goal may never be realized. Instead, genetic therapies may need to be custom-tailored to the individual. Nevertheless, advances in scientific and medical technology may eventually endow us with the ability to provide custom genetic therapy to those in need as easily as we deliver traditional medicine.

References

1. Schenborn ET. Transfection technologies. In: Tymms MJ, ed. Methods in Molecular Biology. vol 130. Totowa: Humana Press Inc, 2000:91-102.
2. Costa GL, Benson JM, Seroogy CM et al. Targeting rare populations of murine antigen-specific T lymphocytes by retroviral transduction for potential application in gene therapy for autoimmune disease. J Immunol 2000; 164(7):3581-3590.
3. Cui Y, Golob J, Kelleher E et al. Targeting transgene expression to antigen-presenting cells derived from lentivirus-transduced engrafting human hematopoetic stem/progenitor cells. Blood 2002; 99(2):399-408.
4. Aiuti A, Slavin S, Memet A et al. Correction of ADA-SCID by stem cell gene therapy combined with nonmyeloablative conditioning. Science 2002; 296(5577):2410-2413.
5. Martin R, McFarland HF. Immunological aspects of experimental allergic encephalomyelitis and multiple sclerosis. Crit Rev Clin Lab Sci 1995; 32(2):121-182.
6. Shaw MK, Lorens JB, Dhawan A et al. Local delivery of interleukin 4 by retrovirus-transduced T lymphocytes ameliorates experimental autoimmune encephalomyelitis. J Exp Med 1997; 185(9):1711-1714.
7. Mathisen PM, Yu M, Johnson JM et al. Treatment of experimental autoimmune encephalomyelitis with genetically modified memory T cells. J Exp Med 1997; 186(1):159-164.
8. Atkinson MA, Leiter EH. The NOD mouse model of type 1 diabetes: As good as it gets? Nat Med 1999; 5(6):601-604.
9. Moritani M, Yoshimoto K, Ii S et al. Prevention of adoptively transferred diabetes in nonobese diabetic mice with IL-10-transduced islet-specific Th1 lymphocytes: A gene therapy model for autoimmune diabetes. J Clin Invest 1996; 98(8):1851-1859.
10. Yamamoto AM, Chernajovsky Y, Lepault F et al. The activity of immunoregulatory T cells mediating active tolerance is potentiated in nonobese diabetic mice by an IL-4-based retroviral gene therapy. J Immunol 2001; 166:4973-4980.
11. Myers LK, Rosloneic EF, Cremer MA et al. Collagen-induced arthritis, an animal model of autoimmunity. Life Sci 1997; 61(19):1861-1878.
12. Bessis N, Boissier M-C, Ferrara P et al. Attenuation of collagen-induced arthritis in mice by treatment with vector cells engineered to secrete interleukin-13. Eur J Immunol 1996; 26:2399-2403.
13. Chernajovsky Y, Adams G, Triantaphyllopoulos K et al. Pathogenic lymphoid cells engineered to express TGF $\beta 1$ ameliorate disease in a collagen-induced arthritis model. Gen Ther 1997; 4(6):553-559.
14. Prud'homme GJ, Piccirillo CA. The inhibitory effects of transforming growth factor-beta-1 (TGF-$\beta 1$) in autoimmune diseases. J Autoimmun 2000; 14:23-42.
15. Nakajima A, Seroogy CM, Sandora MR et al. Antigen-specific T cell-mediated gene therapy in collagen-induced arthritis. J Clin Invest 2001; 107(10):1293-1301.

16. Hammer MH, Schröder G, Risch K et al. Antigen-dependent transgene expression in kidney transplantation: A novel approach using gene-engineered T lymphocytes. J Am Soc Nephrol 2002; 13:511-518.
17. Grill RJ, Blesch A, Tuszynski MH. Robust growth of chronically injured spinal cord axons induced by grafts of genetically modified NGF-secreting cells. Exp Neurol 1997; 148:444-452.
18. Staddon JM, Rubin L. Cell adhesion, cell junctions and the blood-brain barrier. Curr Opin Neurobiol 1996; 6(5):622-627.
19. Schwartz M, Moalem G. Beneficial immune activity after CNS injury: Prospects for vaccination. J Neuroimmunol 2001; 113:185-192.
20. Flügel A, Matsumuro K, Neumann H et al. Anti-inflammatory activity of nerve growth factor in experimental autoimmune encephalomyelitis: Inhibition of monocyte transendothelial migration. Eur J Immunol 2001; 31:11-22.
21. Prineas JW, Graham JS. Multiple sclerosis: Capping of surface immunoglobulin G on macrophages engaged in myelin breakdown. Ann Neurol 1981; 10:149-158.
22. Trapp BD, Peterson J, Ransohoff RM et al. Axonal transection in the lesions of multiple sclerosis. N Engl J Med 1998; 338(5):278-285.
23. Mathisen PM, Johnson JM, Kawzcak JA et al. Differential DM20 gene expression distinguishes two distinct patterns of spontaneous recovery from murine autoimmune encephalomyelitis. J Neurosci Res 2001; 64:542-551.
24. Mathisen PM, Yu M, Yin L et al. Th2 cells expressing transgene PDGF-A serve as vectors for gene therapy in autoimmune demyelinating disease. J Autoimmun 1999; 13:31-38.
25. Chen Y, Rosloniec E, Goral MI et al. Redirection of T cell effector function in vivo and enhanced collagen-induced arthritis mediated by an IL-2Rα/IL-4Rβ chimeric receptor transgene. J Immunol 2001; 166:4163-4169.
26. Lafaille JJ, Van de Keere AL, Hsu AL et al. Myelin basic protein-specific T helper 2 (Th2) cells cause experimental autoimmune encephalomyelitis in immunodeficient hosts rather than protect them from disease. J Exp Med 1997; 186:307-312.
27. Pakala SV, Kurrer MO, Katz JD. T helper 2 (Th2) T cells induce acute pancreatitis and diabetes in immune-compromised nonobese diabetic (NOD) mice. J Exp Med 1997; 186(2):299-306.
28. Matsui Y, Inobe M, Okamoto H et al. Blockade of T cell costimulatory signals using adenovirus vectors prevents both the induction and the progression of experimental autoimmune myocarditis. J Mol Cell Cardiol 2002; 34:279-295.
29. Zhang H, Yang Y, Horton J et al. Amelioration of collagen-induced arthritis by CD95 (Apo-1/Fas)-ligand gene transfer. J Clin Invest 1997; 100(8):1951-1957.
30. Jyothi MD, Flavell R, Geiger TL. Targeting autoantigen-specific T cells and suppression of autoimmune encephalomyelitis with receptor-modified T lymphocytes. Nat Biotechnol 2002; 20(12):1215-1220.
31. Tuohy VK, Yu M, Yin L et al. The epitope spreading cascade during progression of experimental autoimmune encephalomyelitis and multiple sclerosis. Immunol Rev 1998; 164:93-100.
32. Yu M, Johnson JM, Tuohy VK. A predictable sequential determinant spreading cascade invariably accompanies progression of experimental autoimmune encephalomyelitis: A basis for peptide-specific therapy after onset of clinical disease. J Exp Med 1996; 183:1777-1788.
33. Yin L, Yu M, Edling AE et al. Preemptive targeting of the epitope spreading cascade with genetically modified regulatory T cells during autoimmune demyelinating disease. J Immunol 2001; 167:6105-6112.
34. Garren H, Steinman L. DNA vaccination in the treatment of autoimmune disease. In: Fathman CG, ed. Biologic and gene therapy of autoimmune disease. Basel: Karger, 2000:203-216.
35. Ruiz PJ, Garren H, Ruiz IU et al. Suppressive immunization with DNA encoding a self-peptide prevents autoimmune disease: Modulation of T cell costimulation. J Immunol 1999; 162:3336-3341.
36. Tsunoda I, Kuang LQ, Tolley ND et al. Enhancement of experimental autoimmune encephalomyelitis (EAE) by DNA immunization with myelin proteolipid protein (PLP) plasmid DNA. J Neuropathol Exp Neurol 1998; 57:758-767.
37. Chen C-C, Rivera A, Ron N et al. A gene therapy approach for treating T-cell-mediated autoimmune diseases. Blood 2001; 97(4):886-894.

38. Agarwal RK, Kang Y, Zambidis E et al. Retroviral gene therapy with an immunoglobulin-antigen fusion construct protects from experimental autoimmune uveitis. J Clin Invest 2000; 106(2):245-252.
39. Wildbaum G, Youssef S, Karin N. A targeted DNA vaccine augments the natural immune response to self TNF-α and suppresses ongoing adjuvant arthritis. J Immunol 2000; 165:5860-5866.
40. Wildbaum G, Karin N. Augmentation of natural immunity to a pro-inflammatory cytokine (TNF-alpha) by targeted DNA vaccine confers long-lasting resistance to experimental autoimmune encephalomyelitis. Gene Ther 1999; 6(6):1128-1138.
41. Wildbaum G, Netzer N, Karin N. Plasmid DNA encoding IFN-γ-inducible protein 10 redirects antigen-specific T cell polarization and suppresses experimental autoimmune encephalomyelitis. J Immunol 2002; 168:5885-5892.
42. Kessels HWHG, Wolkers MC, van den Boom MD et al. Immunotherapy through TCR gene transfer. Nat Immunol 2001; 2(10):957-961.
43. Croxford JL, Feldmann M, Chernajovsky Y et al. Different therapeutic outcomes in experimental allergic encephalomyelitis dependent upon the mode of delivery of IL-10: A comparison of the effects of protein, adenoviral or retroviral IL-10 delivery into the central nervous system. J Immunol 2001; 166:4124-4130.
44. Morita Y, Yang J, Gupta R et al. Dendritic cells genetically engineered to express IL-4 inhibit murine collagen-induced arthritis. J Clin Invest 2001; 107:1275-1284.
45. Julius MA, Yan Q, Zhang Z et al. Q vectors, bicistronic vectors for gene transfer. Biotechniques 2000; 28(4):702-708.
46. Zhao-Emonet JC, Marodon G, Pioche-Durieu C et al. T cell-specific expression from Mo-MLV retroviral vectors containing a CD4 mini-promoter/enhancer. J Gene Med 2000; 2:416-425.
47. Kaczmarczyk SJ, Green JE. A single vector containing modified cre recombinase and LOX recombination sequences for inducible tissue-specific amplification of gene expression. Nucleic Acids Res 2001; 29(12):e56.
48. Bunting M, Bernstein KE, Greer JM et al. Targeting genes for self-excision in the germ line. Genes Dev 1999; 13:1524-1528.
49. Mullen CA. Metabolic suicide genes in gene therapy. Pharmacol Ther 1994; 63:199-207.
50. Cohen JL, Boyer O, Salomon B et al. Prevention of graft-versus-host disease in mice using a suicide gene expressed in T lymphocytes. Blood 1997; 89(12):4636-4645.
51. Bordignon C, Bonini C, Verzeletti S et al. Transfer of the HSV-tk gene into donor peripheral blood lymphocytes for in vivo modulation of donor anti-tumor immunity after allogeneic bone marrow transplantation. Hum Gen Ther 1995; 6(6):813-819.
52. Thomas-Vaslin V, Bellier B, Cohen JL et al. Prolonged allograft survival through conditional and specific ablation of alloreactive T cells expressing a suicide gene. Transplantation 2000; 69(10):2002-2003.
53. Panitch HS, Hirsch RL, Haley AS et al. Exacerbations of multiple sclerosis in patients treated with gamma interferon. Lancet 1987; 1(8538):893-895.
54. Willard HF. Artificial chromosomes coming to life. Science 2000; 290(5495):1308-1309.
55. Chandler LA, Doukas J, Gonzalez AM et al. FGF2-targeted adenovirus encoding platelet-derived growth factor-B enhances de novo tissue formation. Mol Ther 2000; 2(2):153-160.
56. Ko KS, Lee M, Koh JJ et al. Combined administration of plasmids encoding IL-4 and IL-10 prevents the development of autoimmune diabetes in nonobese diabetic mice. Mol Ther 2001; 4(4):313-316.
57. Matzinger P. Tolerance, danger, and the extended family. Annu Rev Immunol 1994; 12:991-1045.
58. Bach J-F. NonTh2 regulatory T-cell control of Th1 autoimmunity. Scand J Immunol 2001; 54:21-29.
59. Dudley ME, Wunderlich JR, Robbins PF et al. Cancer regression and autoimmunity in patients after clonal repopulation with antitumor lymphocytes. Science 2002; 298(5594):850-854.
60. Cavazzana-Calvo M, Hacien-Bey S, de Saint Basile G et al. Gene therapy of human severe combined immunodeficiency (SCID)-X1 disease. Science 2000; 288(5466):669-672.
61. Sugarman J. Ethical considerations in leaping from bench to bedside. Science 1999; 285(5436):2071-2072.

Chapter 5

Therapeutic Gene Transfer for Rheumatoid Arthritis

Natacha Bessis* and Marie-Christophe Boissier

Introduction

Gene therapy was envisaged originally to cure inherited recessive disorders such as cystic fibrosis. The first true gene therapy success was obtained in 2000[1] at Necker Hospital in Paris by Fischer's group who treated babies with severe combined immunodeficiency X1 (SCID-X), forced to live in tightly-controlled, sterile "bubbles" to avoid threats to their nonexistent immune system. Those patients received the normal gene of the common cytokine receptor γ chain which allowed them to restore immune function and to return to a normal life. Even if two of these children have developed a leukemia 3 years later,[2] those children were cured and doomed to imminent death without the gene therapy.

If gene therapy is logically the best strategy to cure monogenic diseases, it can also give a therapeutic solution to polygenic, multifactorial disorders such as cancers and autoimmune diseases. In those pathologies, gene therapy aims at delivering therapeutic molecules that have proved to play a pivotal role in the physiopathological mechanisms of the targeted disease. Many proteins that are commonly used for autoimmune diseases have short half-lifes (cytokines for instance) necessitating frequent and repetitive injections, and they are expensive to synthetize. Gene therapy offers the mean to overcome these limitations by providing safe and long term protein administration in vivo.

Rheumatoid arthritis (RA) is one of these polygenic, multifactorial diseases. It is a common and severe disease. Its prevalence in adults is about 0.5%. It not only causes joint pain and severe disability but also increases mortality. RA is an inflammatory autoimmune disease whose inciting stimulus is unknown, but the cascade of immunological and inflammatory reactions has been elucidated. These reactions produce inflammatory synovitis promptly followed by irreversible joint and bone destruction.[3] Available treatments for RA fail to provide long-lasting control of the symptoms or disease progression. The beneficial effects of conventional second-line therapy are incomplete and usually short-lived, despite the progress brought by the introduction of methotrexate in the 1980s. Recent improvements in our knowledge of the pathophysiology of RA have led to the development of biological treatments. Recently developed agents for biological therapy fall into two categories: TNF-α inhibitors and IL-1 inhibitors. These biological treatments provide significant efficacy in the short and medium term in many patients.[4-6]

*Natacha Bessis—UPRES EA-3408, Immunology, Université Paris 13, 74 rue Marcel Cachin, Bobigny cedex, France. Email: bessis@smbh.univ-paris13.fr

Gene Therapy of Autoimmune Disease, edited by Gérald J. Prud'homme.

As many non inherited recessive disorders, RA is a good candidate for gene therapy since it is a chronic disease, and that many proteins have been shown to be involved in the pathogenic process and thus are specific therapeutic candidates to RA treatments. The strategy of gene therapy needs to define three parameters:

- the gene encoding the molecule used for its therapeutic effect in RA: for instance, the TNF soluble receptor (sTNFR) the IL-1 receptor antagonist (IL-1Ra);
- the vector to be used to transfer the gene: vectors are frequently viral particles, but may be also of nonviral origin (plasmids, or synthetic vectors);
- the targeted tissue: in RA, the choice is first between systemic administration (intravenous [i.v.] or intramuscular [i.m.]) or local administration (i.e., directly within the joint).

Vectors for Gene Therapy of RA

Several gene delivery systems have been developed during the last decade which include viral and nonviral vectors.[7] Each of the vector strategies has its strengths, as well as weaknesses and differs by its efficiency to deliver a therapeutic gene into a given target tissue.

Nonviral Vectors

Plasmids can be used for gene therapy. They are fragments of DNA of bacterial origin. One of the main advantage of plasmids in gene transfer is they can integrate large exogeneous genes. They are characterized by an excellent safety and low immunogenic properties. These vectors are easy to produce on a large scale for clinical use.[8] They may be transferred to cells by simple injection, but this plain method (naked DNA) is poorly efficient. In gene therapy, plasmids are generaly used combined to an enhancing technology, as follows:

Plasmids and Chemical Technology

Cationic lipids form liposomes spontaneously. Plasmidic DNA can form complexes with these liposomes; this lipoplex is able to penetrate the cell membrane, by endocytosis or fusion of the cell membrane. Actually, experimental protocols with this technique in experimental models of arthritis are only a few,[9] certainly because of the poor efficiency of the method.

Plasmids and Physical Technology Electrotransfer

Electric pulses have been used to introduce foreign DNA into various cell types. This method, called cell electroporation, has been successfully applied to in vivo models. Our group and others recently reported an efficient method for transferring DNA into muscle fibers, in which an intramuscular injection of plasmid DNA is followed by delivery of low-field-strength, long-duration, squarewave electric pulses through external electrodes.[10] Exposure of skeletal muscle to a pulsed electric field increases more than 100-fold the expression of a transgene injected i.m. in mice. Moreover, the number of transfected muscle fibers is also increased by a 10 to 50 fold factor. This electric field-mediated transfection of plasmids encoding a gene of interest, also called electrotransfer, ensures not only a high level of transgene expression in the transfected muscle, but also elevated sustained plasma levels of the protein gene product, which is continuously released into the circulation by the highly vascularized muscle cells. Studies showed the efficiency of this new strategy in experimental models of RA, by electrotransfer of plasmids encoding IL-10,[11] sTNFR,[12,13] and very recently with IL-4[14] or IL-1ra.[15]

Plasmids and Cell Biology

The cell can be considered as a vector. Cultured cells may be used as vectors after transfection. They are able to synthetise and secrete the therapeutic protein, in vitro and in vivo. The transfected cells may be inert or active. If inert, the transfection uses them as biologic protein factories; fibroblasts or keratinocytes can be used in this occurrence. Conversely, the specific activity of the cells to be transfected may be useful in some specific protocols, e.g., for tissue repair or immunomodulation.

Viral Vectors

They are the most often used vectors in clinical protocols of gene therapy. Viruses are employed because of their capacity to integrate DNA fragments and their natural ability to enter the cell, then using the cell machinery to synthesize the proteins encoded by the viral genome. The main advantage of a viral system in gene therapy is the ability to obtain high levels of the therapeutic protein. The main problems encountered with viruses are their immunogenicity (see section *Immunogenicity Induced by Gene Therapy Vectors*) and the integration of the viral genome within the genome of the host. The most used vectors are retroviruses, adenoviruses, and adeno-associated viruses (AAV).

Retroviral and Lentiviral Vectors

Moloney Murine Leukemia Viruses (MoMLV)-derived Retroviral Vectors (RV) are frequently used vectors in gene therapy studies in both animal models and in clinical trials. Stable transgene integration into dividing cells and absence of immune reaction against vector particles are the main advantages of recombinant RV vectors. In early studies of RA, synoviocytes harvested surgically from the joints of animals could easily be transduced ex vivo using even low titers of recombinant RV. Transduced cells expressed the transgene in vitro for at least 5 weeks and this fell rapidly over time.[16] Engraftment of ex vivo transduced syngeneic synoviocytes into rat arthritic joints allowed expression of the transgene for about 2 weeks.[17,18] Human synovial fibroblasts (SF) are also transduced efficiently (>70%) with RV vectors encoding IL1Ra, sTNFRp55 or IL10 resulting in secretion of soluble molecules for at least 60 days in culture conditions. Implantation of the IL1Ra, or IL10 transduced human fibroblast into SCID mice has resulted in reduced perichondrocyte degradation as well as synovial cell invasion.[19] More recently, a similar strategy using retrovirally transduced fibroblasts with a gene encoding a ribozyme targeting matrix metalloproteinase 1 (MMP-1) was shown to reduce RA SF invasiveness in the mouse SCID model.[20]

Direct in vivo transduction of synoviocytes can also be achieved, but only using high-titer RV.[17,21] Transgene expression was transient, declining following injections in rats after 1 week and in rabbits after 4 weeks[16] RV-derived MFG vectors carrying the IL-1Ra gene have been administered locally into joints and systemically into haematopoietic stem cells[22] Although transient (4 to 6 weeks), efficient intra-articular secretion of human IL-1Ra was observed in several animal models of arthritis, exceeding its usually estimated therapeutic level. The MFG-IL-1Ra vectors were used to transduce human synoviocytes in vitro and in two clinical studies for RA.[23]

In contrast to RV-derived vectors, lentivirus-derived vectors enable the stable transduction of both dividing and nondividing cells. Nevertheless, the potential risk of insertional mutations due to integration of additional virus sequences into the human genome is a large concern, and should be further studied before using retroviral or lentiviral vectors in a clinical setting. This new vector has recently been shown to be efficient in transducing human primary synovial fibroblasts; moreover, after intra-articular injection into SCID mice, these transduced cells could efficiently express the transgene in vivo.[24]

Adenoviral Vectors

Recombinant vectors derived from different serotypes of human adenovirus (Ad) have been used extensively in animal models of RA. The host range of the Ad vectors can be changed by modifying the viral fibre proteins so that they can interact more properly with different cell surface components.[25] A dose dependent efficacy has been observed by different groups with concomitant development of synovitis in rabbits,[26] rats,[27] rhesus monkeys,[28] and mice in which transgene expression weakened after the first week of transduction.[29] Ad vectors transduce synoviocytes very efficiently ex vivo. However, their use is hampered by enhanced inflammation in the synovium, limited transgene persistence and difficulty of repeated inoculation (see section *Immunogenicity Induced by Gene Therapy Vectors*) Further improvements in producing higher titers of gutted or weak immunogenic Ad vectors are needed for long-term transgene expression.

Adeno-Associated Virus

The adeno-associated virus (AAV) is a small single stranded DNA virus. Vectors derived from AAV have several properties favorable to their use in gene therapy for rheumatoid arthritis. Their natural innocuousness, wide tropism spectrum,[30] long-term pharmacologically regulable transgene expression[31] and weak immunogenicity are particularly important in the context of a chronic inflammatory disease such as RA. Several studies demonstrated that AAV vectors efficiently transduced synovial cells[32-34] and human primary chondrocytes in vitro.[35] The efficacy of AAV-mediated gene transfer in RA models was evaluated after either direct injection into animal joints or injection into muscle.[36] Recombinant AAV vectors encoding IL4, IL-10, vIL-10, sTNFR and IL1Ra were evaluated in various rodent models of RA. Joint administration in a LPS induced RA rat model showed persistence of the AAV vector. A CMV promoter-mediated inflammation-enhanced transduction of synoviocytes was observed allowing for reactivation of transgene expression.[33] rAAV-IL1Ra administration in this model led to improvement of the biological markers of the disease.[37] Expression of IL-1Ra could be disease-reactivated 80 days after the initial exposure, thus preventing a recurrent arthritic episode. Intramuscular administration of a rAAV encoding IL-4 in the collagen-induced arthritis (CIA) mouse model showed long-term (129 days) IL-4 expression in muscle, and injection within the tarsus improved clinical scores.[36] Intra-articular administration of rAAV in a similar CIA mouse model also demonstrated long-term expression (7 months). Intra-articular injection of rAAV encoding sTNFR1 in a TNF-α transgenic mouse model of RA showed that both synoviocytes and muscle cells were transduced[38] resulting in a noticeable amelioration of the joint score up to 2 months after administration. A disease inducible rAAV transduction was also performed.[34] A recent study showed that, after intra-articular injection of an AAV vector encoding the sTNFR gene, the systemic distribution of the gene product was reduced as compared to systemic injection.[39] This supports interest in the intra-articular route of gene administration in joint disease.

Immunogenicity Induced by Gene Therapy Vectors

Circumventing the immune response to the vector is a major challenge with all vector types (see ref. 40 for an extensive review). Viral vectors are the most likely to induce an immune response, especially those, like adenovirus and AAV, which express immunogenic epitopes within the organism. The first immune response occurring after vector transfer emerges from the innate immune system, mainly consisting in rapid (few hours) inflammatory cytokines and chemokines secretion around the administration site. This reaction is high with adenoviral vectors and almost null with AAV. It is noteworthy that plasmids DNA vectors, because of CpG stimulatory islets, also stimulate innate immunity via the stimulation of TLR receptors on leukocytes. Specific immune responses leading to antibody production and T lymphocyte activation also occur within a few days after vector introduction. Capsid antigens are mostly responsible for specific immunity toward adenoviruses, and are also involved in the response against AAV. In the former case only, however, viral gene-encoded proteins can also be immunogenic. Preexisting humoral immunity resulting from early infections with wild type AAV or adenovirus can prevent efficient gene transfer with the corresponding vector. In all cases, some parameters like the route of administration, dose, or promoter type have been extensively described as critical factors influencing vector immunity. Strategies to prevent vector-induced immunity could come from the immunology field, since tolerance induction or immunosuppression are possibilities. The use of new viral serotypes of either adenovirus or AAV is also a possibility, since not all serotypes induce the same degree of immune response in humans. Alterations to vector structure have also been extensively performed to circumvent the immune system, and thus enhance gene transfer efficiency and safety.

What Are the Best Candidate Genes for Gene Therapy in RA?

The choice should be based on the respective role of the various processes involved in RA (Fig. 1). Several molecules may be used simultaneously. This can be achieved either by using gene therapy to produce several products or by combining gene therapy and conventional biological therapy.

The treatment of an autoimmune disease such as RA should target the triggering autoantigen or the receptor specific for the relevant epitope of that antigen. Unfortunately, this phase of the pathogenesis of RA remains unelucidated. An alternative strategy is to interrupt the cascade set off by the specific antigen stimulus. Gene therapy might achieve this in several ways, for instance by promoting soluble CTLA-4 or CD28 expression[41] to block T-cell activation in response to presentation of the antigen, or by increasing soluble CD40 levels to inhibit B-cell differentiation and block interactions between T cells and B cells.[42,43]

The inflammatory reaction itself is currently the most studied target for biological therapy. IL-1 and TNF-α act in synergy to orchestrate the entire inflammatory process[44] IL-1 can be effectively blocked by IL-1Ra, which binds to the IL-1 receptors, making them unavailable for IL-1.[45] The second IL-1 receptor (IL-1RII) is also an IL-1 inhibitor, because when located on the cell membrane it binds IL-1 but fails to transmit a signal, acting as a decoy receptor,[46] and when soluble, it binds IL-1, decreasing the amount of soluble IL-1 available for binding to the IL-1RI receptor. Targeting IL-1RI would probably be of limited efficacy; in particular blocking this receptor characterized by high affinity for the natural IL-1 inhibitor IL-1Ra, may increase the availability of membrane IL-1RI, thereby increasing transmission of the signal that activates IL-1.[47,48] TNF-α, the other major player in the inflammatory process, can be inhibited by overexpression of one of its receptors, either p55 (type I) or p75 (type II). Thus, an adenovirus containing the gene for the fusion protein sTNFRI/IgG1 inhibits collagen-induced arthritis (CIA) in mice[49-51] and antigen-induced arthritis in rabbits (AIA).[52] The gene encoding the monomeric form of sTNFRII, which is expressed after ex vivo splenocyte infection by a retrovirus, inhibits CIA.[53] Another means of inhibiting inflammation is to increase levels of anti-inflammatory cytokines. IL-4, IL-13, and IL-10 can inhibit the release of pro-inflammatory cytokines and can decrease the production of Th1 cytokines such as interferon-γ.[54-56] This effect is accompanied by increased production of IL-1Ra and enhanced release of Th2 cytokines (self-amplification loop). Viral IL-10 (homologous to IL-10 and encoded by the Epstein-Barr virus), in contrast to mammalian IL-10, has anti-inflammatory effects but causes only minimal immunosuppression.[57-59]

Further downstream along the cascade, the balance between tissue repair and tissue destruction can be altered by modifying metalloproteinase inhibition or growth factors. Growth factors such as BMP-2, IGF-1, FGF, or TGF-β may be useful for repairing cartilage or bone lesions.[60] A major difficulty with biological therapies focused on tissue repair may be timing. The treatment would probably not be useful in the advanced disease, at a stage when the lesions are irreversible.

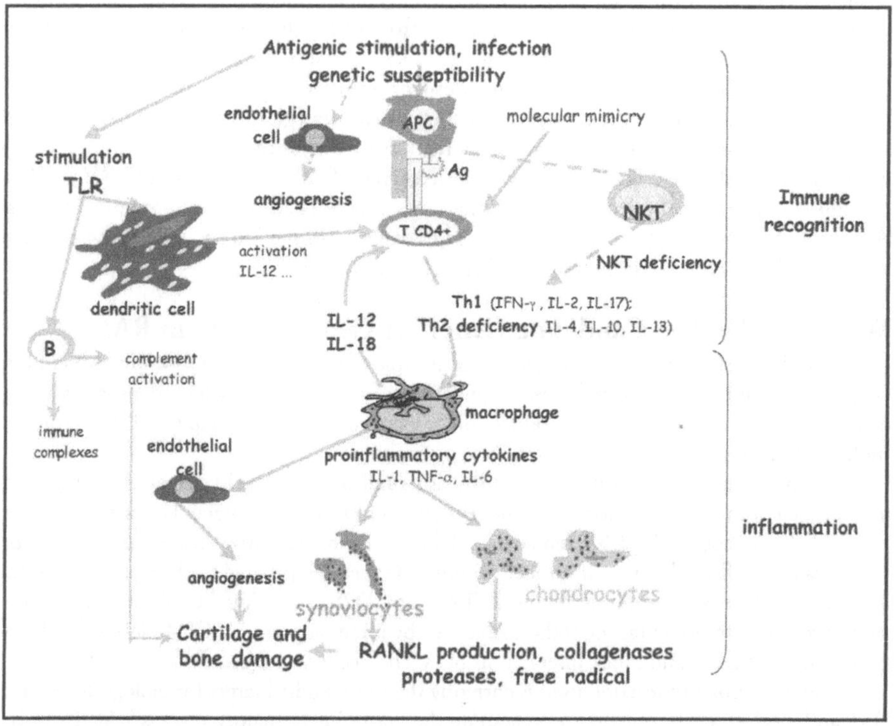

Figure 1. Immunopathogenesis of rheumatoid arthritis. Abbreviations: Ag, antigen; APC, antigen-presenting cell; B, B lymphocyte; NKT, natural killer T cell; RANKL, receptor activator of nuclear factor kappa B ligand; TLR, Toll-like receptor.

It is also possible to achieve synovectomy by gene therapy (gene therapy-mediated synovectomy). The local transfection of synoviocytes by the thymidine kinase gene of herpes simplex virus followed by administration of the prodrug ganciclovir causes lysis of the synoviocytes;[28] the thymidine kinase converts ganciclovir to a nucleotide analogue that blocks the synthesis of DNA, thus destroying dividing cells. An alternative is transfection of the Fas ligand gene, which causes apoptosis of the synoviocytes. Fas gene expression is considerably increased in RA synoviocytes, whereas Fas ligand (FasL) levels are low, resulting in increased survival and in proliferation of these cells within the rheumatoid synovium. FasL concentrations can be upregulated by injecting the corresponding gene into the joint. This method has been shown to induce apoptosis of cultured synovial cells from human rheumatoid membrane[61] and to improve CIA.[62] FasL stimulation can also be achieved by transferring the FADD gene (Fas-associated death domain) into the synovial cells.[63]

How to Choose between Local and Systemic Treatment?

Two different methods could be used in RA. One is local treatment, i.e., injection in or about the joints, and the other is systemic treatment by parenteral injection (intramuscular, intravenous, subcutaneous or, in animals, intraperitoneal). Although flares sometimes predominate in one or two joints, a far more common pattern is polyarticular disease and in some cases extra-articular involvement.[8]

Local treatment seeks to achieve high concentrations of the therapeutic protein within the joint fluid and/or synovial membrane. Most studies have used genes encoding a secreted form of a protein, which is delivered to cells residing in tissues within the joint. A major advantage of this method is that high protein levels can be obtained at the arthritic site. However, systemic effects can occur, in particular as a result of transsynovial diffusion. Soluble molecules easily cross the synovial membrane, which has no basement membrane, and consequently any local articular treatment has the potential to induce systemic effects. It explains why a vector injected into a joint can be found throughout the body. Furthermore, local vector injections may have contralateral effects.[64]

These considerations have led to the development of systemic treatments, which may obviate the need for injecting multiple joints. The rationale for systemic treatment is that RA is a systemic disease whose joint manifestations depend, at least in part, on systemic immune disorders. A theoretical obstacle is that the far greater production of therapeutic protein needed for systemic therapy requires injection of a higher dose of vector, which can be difficult to produce. Furthermore, the higher concentrations in the bloodstream may cause side effects related to the vector and/or to the therapeutic protein. Consequently, development of this strategy is compatible only with models or applications in which efficacy is demonstrated after introduction into the body of a moderate amount of the vector with its therapeutic gene. From a long-term perspective, systemic treatments may prove easier to use.

How to Choose between in Vivo and ex Vivo Strategies?

The goal of gene therapy is to replace conventional biological methods by achieving continuous expression during a given period of time, production and, in most cases, release of a therapeutic protein. Cells capable of expressing the gene of interest are chosen. The gene is introduced into those cells, either ex vivo or in vivo. In this respect, gene therapy follows the same rules in RA as in other polyallelic diseases.

Ex vivo gene transfer was the first method used for gene therapy in arthritis models. Synovial cells are harvested and synovial fibroblasts (type B synovial cells) cultured and infected with a retroviral vector encoding the gene of interest. This gene was IL-1Ra in the earliest studies. After expansion and infection with the vector, the synovial cells are injected into the joints of the donor animals. Thus, this method is similar to autologous grafting. Experiments conducted with IL1-Ra have provided convincing evidence that the IL-1Ra gene is expressed within the synovium of the injected joint and that IL-1Ra is present in the joint fluid. Other cell types can be transfected ex vivo and reinjected into the animal, including myoblasts, skin fibroblasts, T cells, and dendritic cells. Reinjection can be performed at a site other than the joint to achieve systemic therapy of RA. Splenocytes transfected ex vivo by a retrovirus encoding sTNFR or TGF-β1[65] inhibit CIA arthritis in mice. Furthermore, the ex vivo method can be performed with nonretroviral vectors, such as adenoviruses.[51] Plasmid vectors have also been employed successfully. Lines of xenogeneic fibroblasts (Chinese hamster ovary cells) or human keratinocytes have been transfected with plasmids encoding various anti-inflammatory cytokines, and grafted into the subcutaneous tissues of mice with CIA.[54,48] Despite the short lifespan of the cells expressing the therapeutic gene, significant efficacy was found. The cells can be protected by encapsulation into hollow fibres permeable to therapeutic molecules, thus constituting an implantable bioreactor.[56] However, after ex vivo plasmid transfection, autologous skin fibroblasts seem to be the most effective cell type for treating CIA.[66] Finally, the transfected cells used in all these ex vivo methods can be viewed as supervectors that ensure delivery of the therapeutic gene at a selected site. All ex vivo transfection methods allow stringent quality control of gene introduction, good quantitation of transfection efficiency, and control of the site of gene expression prior to reinjection. The difficulty is greatest, however, when ex vivo gene therapy is coupled with a local strategy. The transfected cells injected into the joint are first harvested from a joint (synovial fibroblasts), and the patient must undergo two invasive procedures requiring a high level of accuracy and involving sites that can be hard to access.

In vivo gene transfer is obviously simpler, whether the systemic route or intra-articular injection is used. There is no need to harvest material from the patient or to perform complex manipulations of these cells in the laboratory. However, systemic therapy requires a high vector dose which can be difficult to obtain for some types of vector.

From Preclinical Experiments to Clinical Trials

The evaluation of therapeutic strategies for RA faces a major obstacle, which is the absence of animal models replicating all the aspects of human RA. Available models each replicate one facet of the disease. Consequently, extrapolation of experimental findings to humans requires extreme caution. Overall, available models simulate a RA flare rather than RA itself, which is characterized by flares on a background of chronic disease. Conclusions drawn from experiments should be evaluated in the light of the limitations of a particular model and are not necessarily relevant to other models. All available arthritis models are characterized by a phase of acute or subacute joint inflammation. The degree of joint destruction is variable. Extra-articular manifestations are inconspicuous or receive little attention. Taken in aggregate, animal experiments establish that gene therapy for arthritis is feasible.

The first successful experiments, conducted with transfected fibroblasts or 3T3 cell lines in four different animal models of RA,[17,26,67] prompted a clinical trial in humans with RA. The overall strategy was the same as in the models, i.e., local treatment with reinjection into a joint of synovial cells infected with a retrovirus encoding IL-1Ra. This study, whose protocol is described in detail elsewhere[68] has been completed very recently. The results demonstrate that this gene therapy strategy is feasible in humans. The procedure was extremely cumbersome, however. The clinical study was conducted in patients scheduled for prosthetic replacement of the metacarpophalangeal joints (MCPs). The first step was collection of synovial tissue from a joint. Synovial cells were infected with the MFG-IRAP retrovirus containing cDNA for IL-1Ra, cultured for one week, and prepared for injection into joints other than the donor joint. One week after the injection, the joints were harvested during the MCP replacement procedure. Examination of the joints showed local expression of IL-1Ra. These results prompted similar trials in Europe and the United States.[69]

Future Directions

The active research conducted to improve gene therapy is not specific to rheumatology. Clearly, the various components of gene therapy strategies will have to be noticeably improved before considering routine use in human patients. Intensive research efforts focusing on nonviral vectors have led to the development of electrotransfer, which substantially improves transfection efficiency. Studies on the efficiency of articular electrotransfer are ongoing. The development of synthetic vectors and the amelioration of viral vectors are also a major focus for research.

The selection of genes for transfection has benefited from improvements in our understanding of the biological mechanisms involved in RA. Gene therapy provides access to intracellular molecules, particularly key enzymes or second messengers. In particular, cyclin-dependent kinase inhibitors administered into the joint via adenoviral vectors inhibit synovial proliferation, thus ensuring resolution of arthritis.[70] Similarly, synovial-cell apoptosis can be stimulated by inhibitors of nuclear translocation of nuclear factor-kappaB (NF-κB) transferred via an adenoviral vector.[38] The ability to regulate the release of the protein of interest is another advantage that, in theory, is specific of gene therapy. Most of the transgenes used to date are expressed under the control of viral promoters that are not amenable to regulation. In the treatment of inflammation related to joint destruction, the benefits of the anti-inflammatory effect should be weighed against the potential risks related to presence in the body of anti-inflammatory molecules in high levels (risks of immunosuppression, for instance). Gene expression can be regulated by exogenous molecules (tetracyclines, for example) acting on transgene promoters. Other more subtle strategies are conceivable. An example is self-regulation of the transgene by the inflammation itself. Very recent investigations have shown that intra-articular IL-1Ra gene delivery can be regulated by using the promoter naturally controlling the gene of C3 inflammation protein. Moreover, this strategy was found to prevent CIA in mice.[71] The multiplicity of the factors involved in RA suggests that several molecules used in combination may be more effective than a single molecule. For instance, vIL-10 was shown to synergize with sTNFRI, and sIL-1R also synergizes with sTNFR to inhibit arthritis.[72]

Decreasing the vector's immunogenicity is also a major challenge in the very near future. Elimination of viral epitopes by viral capsid modifications, use of nonimmunogenic virus serotypes and suppression of viral genes from the vector's genome are the most promising strategies experienced until now. Taken together, published studies have firmly established the scientific validity of gene therapy in RA models. Nevertheless, advances are needed to define the reference strategy. To this end, further experimental and preclinical studies must be conducted.

Conclusions

In RA, which is both a polyarticular and a systemic disease, anti-TNF or anti-IL-1 targeted treatment will not be the only solutions proposed to patients in the future. Gene therapy approaches, when introduced, do not imply the exclusion of former therapies. They are only specific and promising examples of targeted therapies that are not based on the use of protein anymore, but rather on a gene encoding this protein. In the future, we will try to achieve a control of the gene expression, just as we tried in the past to control the protein administration in a biotherapy context (frequency of injection, dose of administered protein etc.). In the next few years, the challenges in the gene therapy of RA will be to improve the benefit to risk ratio of vector application, to achieve controlled gene expression, and to elucidate the immune consequences of transgene and vector administration. These parameters are essential and absolutely prerequired to pursue or enter upon any gene therapy clinical trials in patients suffering from rheumatoid arthritis.

Acknowledgments

The work conducted by the authors of this review is supported by the Association de Recherche sur la Polyarthrite (ARP), the Société Française de Rhumatologie (SFR), the Ministère de la Recherche et de la Technologie. Vectors used in a part of the experiments have been provided by the Gene Vector Production Network, funded by Association française contre les myopathies (AFM).

References

1. Cavazzana-Calvo M, Hacein-Bey S, de Saint Basile G et al. Gene therapy of human severe combined immunodeficiency (SCID)-X1 disease. Science 2000; 288:669-672.
2. Hacein-Bey-Abina S, von Kalle C, Schmidt M et al. A serious adverse event after successful gene therapy for X-linked severe combined immunodeficiency. N Engl J Med 2003; 348:255-256.
3. Kavanaugh AFLP. In: Gallin JI, Snyderman R, eds. Rheumatoid arthritis. 3rd ed. Lippincott Williams and Wilkins, 1999:1017-1037.
4. Elliott MJ, Maini RN, Feldmann M et al. Randomised double-blind comparison of chimeric monoclonal antibody to tumour necrosis factor alpha (cA2) versus placebo in rheumatoid arthritis. Lancet 1994; 344:1105-1110.

5. Moreland LW, Baumgartner SW, Schiff MH et al. Treatment of rheumatoid arthritis with a recombinant human tumor necrosis factor receptor (p75)-Fc fusion protein. N Engl J Med 1997; 337:141-147.
6. Campion GV, Lebsack ME, Lookabaugh J et al. Dose-range and dose-frequency study of recombinant human interleukin-1 receptor antagonist in patients with rheumatoid arthritis. The IL-1Ra Arthritis Study Group. Arthritis Rheum 1996; 39:1092-1101.
7. Bessis N, Doucet C, Cottard V et al. Gene therapy in rheumatoid arthritis. J Gene Med 2002; 4:581-591.
8. Ghivizzani SC, Oligino TJ, Glorioso JC et al. Gene therapy approaches for treating rheumatoid arthritis. Clin Orthop 2000; S288-299.
9. Fellowes R, Etheridge CJ, Coade S et al. Amelioration of established collagen induced arthritis by systemic IL-10 gene delivery. Gene Ther 2000; 7:967-977.
10. Bloquel C, Fabre E, Bureau MF et al. Plasmid DNA electrotransfer for intracellular and secreted proteins expression: New methodological developments and applications. J Gene Med 2004; (6 Suppl 1):S11-23.
11. Saidenberg-Kermanach N, Bessis N, Deleuze V et al. Efficacy of interleukin-10 gene electrotransfer into skeletal muscle in mice with collagen-induced arthritis. J Gene Med 2003; 5:164-171.
12. Bloquel C, Bessis N, Boissier MC et al. Gene therapy of collagen-induced arthritis by electrotransfer of human tumor necrosis factor-alpha soluble receptor I variants. Hum Gene Ther 2004; 15:189-201.
13. Kim JM, Ho SH, Hahn W et al. Electro-gene therapy of collagen-induced arthritis by using an expression plasmid for the soluble p75 tumor necrosis factor receptor-Fc fusion protein. Gene Ther 2003; 10:1216-1224.
14. Ho SH, Hahn W, Lee HJ et al. Protection against collagen-induced arthritis by electrotransfer of an expression plasmid for the interleukin-4. Biochem Biophys Res Commun 2004; 321:759-766.
15. Jeong JG, Kim JM, Ho SH et al. Electrotransfer of human IL-1Ra into skeletal muscles reduces the incidence of murine collagen-induced arthritis. J Gene Med 2004; 6:1125-1133.
16. Ghivizzani SC, Lechman ER, Tio C et al. Direct retrovirus-mediated gene transfer to the synovium of the rabbit knee: Implications for arthritis gene therapy. Gene Ther 1997; 4:977-982.
17. Makarov SS, Olsen JC, Johnston WN et al. Retrovirus mediated in vivo gene transfer to synovium in bacterial cell wall-induced arthritis in rats. Gene Ther 1995; 2:424-428.
18. Makarov SS, Olsen JC, Johnston WN et al. Suppression of experimental arthritis by gene transfer of interleukin 1 receptor antagonist cDNA. Proc Natl Acad Sci USA 1996; 93:402-406.
19. Pap T, Gay RE, Gay S. Gene transfer: From concept to therapy. Curr Opin Rheumatol 2000; 12:205-210.
20. Rutkauskaite E, Zacharias W, Schedel J et al. Ribozymes that inhibit the production of matrix metalloproteinase 1 reduce the invasiveness of rheumatoid arthritis synovial fibroblasts. Arthritis Rheum 2004; 50:1448-1456.
21. Bandara G, Mueller GM, Galea-Lauri J et al. Intraarticular expression of biologically active interleukin 1-receptor-antagonist protein by ex vivo gene transfer. Proc Natl Acad Sci USA 1993; 90:10764-10768.
22. Evans CH, Ghivizzani SC, Smith P et al. Using gene therapy to protect and restore cartilage. Clin Orthop 2000; S214-219.
23. Gouze E, Ghivizzani SC, Palmer GD et al. Gene therapy for rheumatoid arthritis. Expert Opin Biol Ther 2001; 1:971-978.
24. Lin YL, Noel D, Mettling C et al. Feline immunodeficiency virus vectors for efficient transduction of primary human synoviocytes: Application to an original model of rheumatoid arthritis. Hum Gene Ther 2004; 15:588-596.
25. Wickham TJ. Targeting adenovirus. Gene Ther 2000; 7:110-114.
26. Otani K, Nita I, Macaulay W et al. Suppression of antigen-induced arthritis in rabbits by ex vivo gene therapy. J Immunol 1996; 156:3558-3562.
27. Evans CH, Ghivizzani SC, Oligino TA et al. Future of adenoviruses in the gene therapy of arthritis. Arthritis Res 2001; 3:142-146.
28. Goossens PH, Schouten GJ, 't Hart B et al. Feasibility of adenovirus-mediated nonsurgical synovectomy in collagen-induced arthritis-affected rhesus monkeys. Hum Gene Ther 1999; 10:1139-1149.

29. Sawchuk SJ, Boivin GP, Duwel LE et al. Anti-T cell receptor monoclonal antibody prolongs transgene expression following adenovirus-mediated in vivo gene transfer to mouse synovium. Hum Gene Ther 1996; 7:499-506.
30. Jomary C, Vincent KA, Grist J et al. Rescue of photoreceptor function by AAV-mediated gene transfer in a mouse model of inherited retinal degeneration. Gene Ther 1997; 4:683-690.
31. Haberman RP, McCown TJ, Samulski RJ. Inducible long-term gene expression in brain with adeno-associated virus gene transfer. Gene Ther 1998; 5:1604-1611.
32. Zhang L, Wang D, Fischer H et al. Efficient expression of CFTR function with adeno-associated virus vectors that carry shortened CFTR genes. Proc Natl Acad Sci USA 1998; 95:10158-10163.
33. Pan RY, Xiao X, Chen SL et al. Disease-inducible transgene expression from a recombinant adeno-associated virus vector in a rat arthritis model. J Virol 1999; 73:3410-3417.
34. Goater J, Muller R, Kollias G et al. Empirical advantages of adeno associated viral vectors in vivo gene therapy for arthritis. J Rheumatol 2000; 27:983-989.
35. Arai Y, Kubo T, Fushiki S et al. Gene delivery to human chondrocytes by an adeno associated virus vector. J Rheumatol 2000; 27:979-982.
36. Cottard V, Mulleman D, Bouille P et al. Adeno-associated virus-mediated delivery of IL-4 prevents collagen-induced arthritis. Gene Ther 2000; 7:1930-1939.
37. Pan RY, Chen SL, Xiao X et al. Therapy and prevention of arthritis by recombinant adeno-associated virus vector with delivery of interleukin-1 receptor antagonist. Arthritis Rheum 2000; 43:289-297.
38. Zhang HG, Huang N, Liu D et al. Gene therapy that inhibits nuclear translocation of nuclear factor kappaB results in tumor necrosis factor alpha-induced apoptosis of human synovial fibroblasts. Arthritis Rheum 2000; 43:1094-1105.
39. Chan JM, Villarreal G, Jin WW et al. Intraarticular gene transfer of TNFR:Fc suppresses experimental arthritis with reduced systemic distribution of the gene product. Mol Ther 2002; 6:727-736.
40. Bessis N, GarciaCozar FJ, Boissier MC. Immune responses to gene therapy vectors: Influence on vector function and effector mechanisms. Gene Ther 2004; 11(Suppl 1):S10-17.
41. Finck BK, Linsley PS, Wofsy D. Treatment of murine lupus with CTLA4Ig. Science 1994; 265:1225-1227.
42. Durie FH, Fava RA, Foy TM et al. Prevention of collagen-induced arthritis with an antibody to gp39, the ligand for CD40. Science 1993; 261:1328-1330.
43. Durie FH, Foy TM, Noelle RJ. The role of CD40 and its ligand (gp39) in peripheral and central tolerance and its contribution to autoimmune disease. Res Immunol 1994; 145:200-205, discussion 244-209.
44. Dayer JM. The saga of the discovery of IL-1 and TNF and their specific inhibitors in the pathogenesis and treatment of rheumatoid arthritis. Joint Bone Spine 2002; 69:123-132.
45. Boissier MC, Bessis N, Falgarone G. Options for blocking interleukin-1 in rheumatoid arthritis. Joint Bone Spine 2002; In press.
46. Colotta F, Re F, Muzio M et al. Interleukin-1 type II receptor: A decoy target for IL-1 that is regulated by IL-4. Science 1993; 261:472-475.
47. Burger D, Chicheportiche R, Giri JG et al. The inhibitory activity of human interleukin-1 receptor antagonist is enhanced by type II interleukin-1 soluble receptor and hindered by type I interleukin-1 soluble receptor. J Clin Invest 1995; 96:38-41.
48. Bessis N, Guery L, Mantovani A et al. The type II decoy receptor of IL-1 inhibits murine collagen-induced arthritis. Eur J Immunol 2000; 30:867-875.
49. Quattrocchi E, Walmsley M, Browne K et al. Paradoxical effects of adenovirus-mediated blockade of TNF activity in murine collagen-induced arthritis. J Immunol 1999; 163:1000-1009.
50. Le CH, Nicolson AG, Morales A et al. Suppression of collagen-induced arthritis through adenovirus-mediated transfer of a modified tumor necrosis factor alpha receptor gene. Arthritis Rheum 1997; 40:1662-1669.
51. Kim SH, Evans CH, Kim S et al. Gene therapy for established murine collagen-induced arthritis by local and systemic adenovirus-mediated delivery of interleukin-4. Arthritis Res 2000; 2:293-302.
52. Oligino T, Ghivizzani S, Wolfe D et al. Intra-articular delivery of a herpes simplex virus IL-1Ra gene vector reduces inflammation in a rabbit model of arthritis. Gene Ther 1999; 6:1713-1720.

53. Chernajovsky Y, Adams G, Podhajcer OL et al. Inhibition of transfer of collagen-induced arthritis into SCID mice by ex vivo infection of spleen cells with retroviruses expressing soluble tumor necrosis factor receptor. Gene Ther 1995; 2:731-735.
54. Bessis N, Boissier MC, Ferrara P et al. Attenuation of collagen-induced arthritis in mice by treatment with vector cells engineered to secrete interleukin-13. Eur J Immunol 1996; 26:2399-2403.
55. Bessis N, Chiocchia G, Kollias G et al. Modulation of proinflammatory cytokine production in tumour necrosis factor-alpha (TNF-alpha)-transgenic mice by treatment with cells engineered to secrete IL-4, IL-10 or IL-13. Clin Exp Immunol 1998; 111:391-396.
56. Bessis N, Honiger J, Damotte D et al. Encapsulation in hollow fibres of xenogeneic cells engineered to secrete IL-4 or IL-13 ameliorates murine collagen-induced arthritis (CIA). Clin Exp Immunol 1999; 117:376-382.
57. Apparailly F, Verwaerde C, Jacquet C et al. Adenovirus mediated transfer of viral IL-10 gene inhibits collagen-induced arthritis. J Immunol 1998; 160:5213-5220.
58. Lechman ER, Jaffurs D, Ghivizzani SC et al. Direct adenoviral gene transfer of viral IL-10 to rabbit knees with experimental arthritis ameliorates disease in both injected and contralateral control knees. J Immunol 1999; 163:2202-2208.
59. Whalen JD, Lechman EL, Carlos CA et al. Adenoviral transfer of the viral IL-10 gene periarticularly to mouse paws suppresses development of collagen-induced arthritis in both injected and uninjected paws. J Immunol 1999; 162:3625-3632.
60. Trippel SB. Growth factor actions on articular cartilage. J Rheumatol Suppl 1995; 43:129-132.
61. Okamoto K, Asahara H, Kobayashi T et al. Induction of apoptosis in the rheumatoid synovium by Fas ligand gene transfer. Gene Ther 1998; 5:331-338.
62. Zhang H, Yang Y, Horton JL et al. Amelioration of collagen-induced arthritis by CD95 (Apo-1/Fas)-ligand gene transfer. J Clin Invest 1997; 100:1951-1957.
63. Kobayashi T, Okamoto K, Kobata T et al. Novel gene therapy for rheumatoid arthritis by FADD gene transfer: Induction of apoptosis of rheumatoid synoviocytes but not chondrocytes. Gene Ther 2000; 7:527-533.
64. Kim SH, Kim S, Evans CH et al. Effective treatment of established murine collagen-induced arthritis by systemic administration of dendritic cells genetically modified to express IL-4. J Immunol 2001; 166:3499-3505.
65. Chernajovsky Y, Adams G, Triantaphyllopoulos K et al. Pathogenic lymphoid cells engineered to express TGF beta 1 ameliorate disease in a collagen-induced arthritis model. Gene Ther 1997; 4:553-559.
66. Bessis N, Cottard V, Saidenberg-Kermanach' N et al. Syngeneic fibroblasts transfected with a plasmid encoding interleukin-4 as nonviral vectors for anti-inflammatory gene therapy in collagen-induced arthritis. J Gene Med 2002; 4:300-307.
67. Bakker AC, Joosten LA, Arntz OJ et al. Prevention of murine collagen-induced arthritis in the knee and ipsilateral paw by local expression of human interleukin-1 receptor antagonist protein in the knee. Arthritis Rheum 1997; 40:893-900.
68. Evans CH, Robbins PD, Ghivizzani SC et al.Clinical trial to assess the safety, feasibility, and efficacy of transferring a potentially anti-arthritic cytokine gene to human joints with rheumatoid arthritis. Hum Gene Ther 1996; 7:1261-1280.
69. Baragi VM. MFG-IRAP University of pittsburgh. Curr Opin Investig Drugs 2000; 1:194-198.
70. Taniguchi K, Kohsaka H, Inoue N et al. Induction of the p16INK4a senescence gene as a new therapeutic strategy for the treatment of rheumatoid arthritis. Nat Med 1999; 5:760-767.
71. Bakker A, van de Loo FAJ, Bennink M et al. Inflammation-inducible intra-articular production of human IL-1 receptor antagonist results in a more efficient inhibition of collagen-induced arthritis than does constitutive expression of the same transgene. Arthritis res 2001; 3(suppl 1):A2.
72. Ghivizzani SC, Lechman ER, Kang R et al. Direct adenovirus-mediated gene transfer of interleukin-1 and tumor necrosis factor alpha soluble receptors to rabbit knees with experimental arthritis has local and distal anti-arthritic effects. Proc Natl Acad Sci USA 1998; 95:4613-4618.

CHAPTER 6

Gene Therapy-Based Approach for Immune Tolerance Induction Using Recombinant Immunoglobulin Carriers

Moustapha El-Amine, Mary Litzinger, Marco E.F. Melo and David W. Scott*

Introduction

The mechanisms of tolerance induction and its breakdown are important to explore because of its involvement in the pathogenesis of many known autoimmune diseases. Tolerance to "self" is not absolute and can be overcome by the immune system after a foreign stimuli caused by pathogens, allergens or other unknown immune errors (e.g., defects in apoptosis) that affect the immune system, causing a switch from tolerance to an immune response. Therefore, autoimmune diseases may often result from an aberrant or dysfunctional immune response that can no longer discriminate between "self" and "non self" proteins. This deregulation will eventually lead to a systemic disease manifested by organ or tissue specific disorder and pathogenesis. Reversal of this breakdown by the re-introduction of tolerance is therefore an important goal.

Laboratories around the globe have tried to use different gene therapy based approaches to modulate the immune response. By definition, gene therapy is based on the introduction of a DNA fragment, expressing a gene or part of a gene, into a host cell in order to reverse, replace, amplify or correct its function. For example, cytokines, receptors or inhibitors have been used by gene therapy to shift the immune response from a TH1 to a TH2 response[1-3] or vice-versa depending on the immune model. Replacement of genes involved in cell death has been used to trigger apoptosis in inflammatory joints of animal models. Immunomodulators such as CTLA-4 fused to an immunoglobulin to increase its half-life have been used in several gene therapy protocols to down regulate the manifestation of autoimmunity in animal models.[4,5] Our lab, for example, has employed retroviral gene transfer into B cells of an immunoglobulin construct carrying major immunodominant peptides or full-length antigens to re-educate the immune system into tolerance induction.[6-11]

Like many other approaches, gene therapy has its own drawbacks that can only be minimized with continuous experimentation and our knowledge of the immune system and molecular biology techniques. One major problem of gene therapy is the vehicle of delivery. Most laboratories use attenuated viruses (adeno-, retro-, lentiviruses etc.) as tools for delivery of the targeted genetic material. These obviously may incur adverse effects in humans because of their

*David W. Scott—Department of Immunology, Jerome Holland Laboratory, American Red Cross, 15601 Crabbs Branch Way, Rockville, Maryland 20855, U.S.A. Email: ScottD@usa.redcross.org

Gene Therapy of Autoimmune Disease, edited by Gérald J. Prud'homme. ©2005 Eurekah.com and Kluwer Academic / Plenum Publishers.

immunogenicity, problems with retroviral insertions and recombination concerns. Thus, they can complicate other health related issues that makes this avenue difficult to employ and gain acceptance by the public in coming years. Another method of gene delivery is "naked DNA" injection. This simple technique is based on the injection of the genetic material without any vehicle of transportation. Scientists rely on the simple principle of endocytosis and DNA delivery to the nucleus through processing cytoplasmic protein carriers. The problem in this approach is the low efficiency of transfer and the triggering of non-specific immune responses due to CpG sequences present in most vectors that can prevent the host cells from expressing the gene. Finally, the use of liposomes is another way of introducing new genes into a host. This technique takes advantage of the lipid bilayer fusion by encapsulating the DNA in a lipid micelle that protects it from phagocytes and insures its safe delivery to the cytoplasm. Different labs have varying levels of success using this approach; perhaps due to the limited knowledge we have about the mechanisms, molecules and lipids involved in this process. In our opinion, this is still a very promising approach that needs to be explored further because of its safety and efficiency in delivery.

In this chapter we will explore the history of the hapten–carrier theory that led to the discovery of the Ig-peptide carriers as mediators of immune tolerance in animal models. Based on the authors' work and in order to understand the principle of tolerogenicity by this system, B-cell antigen presentation and Ig-peptide mechanisms will be revisited. We will re-evaluate published data showing that this gene therapy approach is efficacious in three autoimmune models, which can be adjusted for future clinical trials in human subjects.

Hapten-Carriers in the History of Tolerance

Our laboratory has been studying the effect of immunoglobulin carriers on tolerance induction based on the previous work of several labs, including those of Weigle, Borel and Scott.[12-15] Their work on this subject showed that the use of carriers such as gamma globulins could induce tolerance in host animals. But there were some differences on the fate of B cells among groups. The studies generated by Venkataraman and Scott and their colleagues, showed persistence of the unresponsive (anergic) cells in the spleen by the usage of fluorescein (FITC)-tagged gamma globulin. Those cells disappeared from the spleen in few days if the mice were not challenged with the tolerogen. In mice rechallenged with the tolerogen, antigen-binding cells (ABC) re-appeared in the spleen. Later studies determined those tolerant cells as being B cells that were anergic and cell cycle arrested. On the other hand, Borel and Aldo-Benson's work using a similar system in which DNP was coupled to an isologous murine IgG, showed that unresponsiveness in host animals as well as ABC persisted in the periphery for several weeks. The main difference between the two groups was the use of heterologous IgG in Scott's group versus an isologous IgG in Borel's group. This difference enhanced the hypothesis that carriers play a role in modulating the immune response. Further efforts to elucidate the mechanisms of tolerance induction by hapten-carriers did not progress until the emergence of recombinant DNA technologies.

In 1996, Zambidis et al[7] created transgenic mice that expressed and secreted an IgG_1 fusion protein containing a peptide, p12-26 of the bacteriophage λ cI repressor protein at its N-terminus. This is a full-length immunoglobulin with its heavy chain and Fc portion, unlike fusion protein such as Ig-CTLA-4 or Ig-IL-4 that has only the Fc portion of the protein to enhance the half-life of the carried gene. The p12-26 peptide was chosen for this construct because it contained both a B cell and T cell epitope from the λ cI repressor protein domain, p1-102. This protein was well characterized and the immunodominant epitopes were well known in different strains of mice with different MHC class II haplotypes. The peptide p12-26 is the major immunodominant epitope in $H\text{-}2^d$ mice, whereas $H\text{-}2^b$ mice recognize a more C-terminal peptide, p73-88. Studies on the p12-26-IgG transgenic mice showed high levels of serum peptide IgG fusion protein. These transgenic mice showed extensive unresponsiveness to a challenge with p12-26 or even p1-102. Moreover, Balb/c mice adoptively transferred with transgenic resting or even LPS blasted

B cells or bone marrow cells were also rendered unresponsive to challenge with p12-26. Tolerance could even be transferred with less than 100,000 purified B cells! Together with recombinant DNA technologies, this tolerance induction to p12-26 peptide opened the door for extensive studies to understand the nature of this response.

Further studies by Zaghouani's labs[16] utilized IgG carriers engineered to contain immunodominant epitopes involved in Experimental Autoimmune Encephalomyelitis (EAE). This group demonstrated that their IgG chimeras carrying an encephalitogenic proteolipid peptide 139-151 (Ig-PLP 139-151) induced neonatal tolerance to EAE. Although their system requires neonatal delivery of the carrier, the end result is always suppression of the immune reaction against the specific antigen and reversal of the adverse immune response. While mechanism of action in this system is not clear, it involves cytokine modulation in the lymph node and spleen for tolerance induction.[16]

Gene Transfer of IgG-Peptides

Following the success of the transgenic mice in inducing tolerance, many questions emerged about the nature of this tolerance induction. Clearly in transgenic mice, we cannot distinguish between the induction of neonatal tolerance, meaning that during neonatal development the immune system learned not to attack the fusion protein (i.e., p12-26-IgG) and the maintenance of peripheral tolerance in adults. One method by which this question could be answered is through the emerging gene therapy techniques using replication deficient viruses and transfer into immunocompetent adults. The obvious choice of Zambidis et al[8] were retroviruses, due to their nature of infection (i.e., infecting only dividing cells), their low immunogenicity in mice and their ease of use. A retroviral vector based on Hozumi's retroviral vector used to infect stem cells[17] was engineered (Fig. 1) to contain viral LTR promoters, a β-Actin promoter to control the transcription of the inserted gene and the murine IgG_1 heavy chain in which peptides and antigens will be inserted. The idea of transferring only the heavy chain was to take advantage of the assembly machinery of B cells, which will provide the light chains needed to assemble the molecule and produce a complete immunoglobulin with a peptide on its N-terminus. To establish immune tolerance that mimics the transgenic mice described above, initially bone marrow from adult mice were cultured ex vivo for two days with the engineered retrovirus and cytokines, and then adoptively transferred to sub-lethally irradiated mice. Continuous serum level of the fusion protein was monitored using NIP-binding ELISAs since the IgG heavy chain had high affinity for that hapten. Two months later, when the immune system had recovered, those mice were challenged with p12-26 and p1-102 and shown to be unresponsive to both at cellular and humoral levels. RT-PCRs were performed to demonstrate the persistence of the gene in the spleen and marrow of tolerant (versus control) mice. This experiment proved that the transgenic model was valid but also convinced the

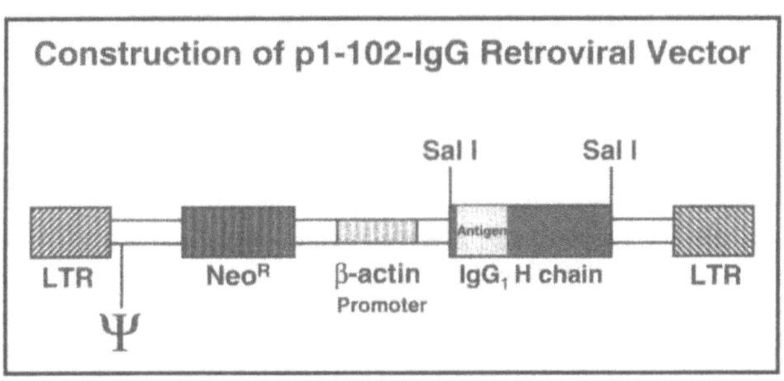

Figure 1. MBAE retroviral construct used for tolerance studies. The vector is engineered with a murine IgG1 heavy chain cassette designed to carry a variety of antigens and peptides on its N terminus. The gene is driven by a β-Actin promoter. The retrovirus insertion and assembly are empowered by LTR.

group to pursue gene therapy as a better approach to understand tolerance induction by IgG-peptides. Subsequently, experiments were successfully performed using infected and LPS-activated B cells that showed tolerance induction in host mice. This latter experiment showed the potential of using this approach in a clinical setting using drawn blood from affected patients to which an autoantigen will be transferred on the tip of the IgG to re-educate the immune system and induce tolerance to several autoimmune diseases, such as juvenile diabetes, uveitis, multiple sclerosis and possibly others such as lupus or rheumatoid arthritis (cf. 10, 11). In order to achieve this goal, an elucidation of the mechanisms of action behind this tolerance induction was needed.

Following those experiments, several questions arose, such as: which is more important to achieve tolerance, secretion or presentation of the IgG-peptide? Are B cells required to present or can any other APC lead to tolerance? What is the role of suppressive cytokines, such as IL-10? Does this tolerance follow the classic signal 1 – signal 2 activation model? If yes, is CTLA-4 involved or not? Can this system induce tolerance to primed animals, which would mimic an autoimmune patient with elevated titers of anti-self antibodies or primed T-cell clones? What are the roles of Fc receptors and the requirement for the Fc portion of the immunoglobulin in the construct? Can different modulators or activators of the immune system such as CD40, Flt3L or CpG sequences be used to activate the B cells and affect the outcome of tolerance? Finally, can this model be applied on animal models of known human autoimmune diseases?

Mechanism of Action

Role of the IgG Carrier, Fc Receptors, and MHC Class II in Tolerance

To answer the questions mentioned in the previous paragraph, experiments using different animal models lacking or over-expressing some key genes were used. In 1998, our colleague Yubin Kang studied the impact of the immunoglobulin carrier on tolerance induction by infecting bone marrow or activated B cells with vectors for p1-102-IgG or p1-102 alone.[9] Cytokine secretion measured after an in vitro stimulation of splenocytes and lymph node lymphocytes showed a more significant decrease in TH1 and TH2 T cell activities versus the group receiving p1-102 alone, although tolerance did not require the IgG. Thus, while the IgG carrier was not necessary for the induction of tolerance, its presence led to more significant unresponsiveness. Importantly, upon challenge for a secondary response, they found that tolerance was lost with p1-102 alone but persisted with the IgG carrier. It is notable also that the gene persisted in the spleens of host mice for several months after the transfer with both constructs. Thus, they drew the conclusion that IgG_1 as a carrier was necessary for the long-term maintenance of hyporesponsiveness in host mice at both the cellular and humoral levels.

In light of this study, we (El-Amine et al) studied the role of the Fc portion on tolerance induced by IgG-peptide constructs.[18] To do this, we used different FcR KO mice both as hosts and as donors of the infected B cells. Thus, we found that the presence of FcR was not required for tolerance in this model as the same degree of unresponsiveness was found with FcR negative B cells used either for donor B cells or for both donor and recipients. Thus, although the IgG appeared important in tolerance, FcR do not appear to be involved in this model of tolerance. To formally exclude the Fc portion of the IgG carrier, we also mutated the IgG_1 in the p12-26-IgG construct in position 297 of the Fc region of the heavy chain; this residue controls the ability of IgG to bind to Fc receptors, but also to fix complement and transit tissues.[19] This did not affect the tolerogenicity of the construct. Therefore, both FcR and the biologic function of the Fc portion of the immunoglobulin carrier do not appear to be required for the induction of tolerance. Finally, the injection of anti-FcR antibodies (2.4G2) into host mice that received activated splenocytes from the transgenic mice did not affect tolerance induction. This study also suggests that secretion of the IgG carrier and its uptake by the FcR, for possible presentation by MHC class II molecules, is not the major route for IgG-peptide mediated tolerance. These results show that while neither the Fc nor the FcR are involved in this tolerance, they could be important in the persistence of the tolerance.

The authors also studied the effect of presentation on tolerance induction to compare it with the secretion-uptake hypothesis. In their studies, this group aimed to understand the importance of B cells as antigen presenting cells (APC) in the process of endogenous uptake and presentation on their MHCs of different epitopes of the IgG-carrier molecule. This mode of presentation would then lead to a tolerogenic signal delivered by B cells to specific T cells. In principle, tolerogenic epitopes could then re-educate the immune system to down regulate its response against an autoimmune antigen. To test this hypothesis, we used MHC class II KO mice as donors of bone marrow or B cells. We infected them with the retrovirus containing the IgG-peptide construct and injected them into syngeneic class II positive mice. In this model, B cells transferred with gene will lack the capability of presenting the epitopes encoded therein. Since secretion appears to be a minor route for tolerance induction, an immune response to the peptide in the recipients of MHC class II KO B cells would indicate a major requirement of MHC class II on presenting B cells in this model of tolerance induction. Upon challenge, the immune responses at cellular and humoral levels showed that tolerance was not induced unless class II positive cells were used to present the targeted epitopes.[20] While it is still possible that local uptake of a secreted IgG fusion protein may occur (and the B cells making it would have a selective advantage), class II is necessary on the presenting cells and cross-presentation by host B cells is not involved.

The Scott lab previously used SCID mice as bone marrow donors to test the role of B cells in our gene therapy model, and found tolerance in terms of the primary response.[8] However, since SCID mice (especially older donors) can be "leaky", this hypothesis was re-investigated using B–cell knockout mice (μMT),[20] which we have backcrossed to H-2^{d}. These studies made using μMT (B cell KO) bone marrow infected with the retrovirus demonstrated that B cells were indeed required for tolerance. Thus, these mice have other potential antigen-presenting cells (such as dendritic cells), but lack B cells as APCs. The lack of tolerance in the treated group proved the need for B cells to process and present epitopes and induce tolerance. These experiments shed light on the importance of presentation in this model rather than secretion and uptake (Fig. 2). These results suggest that B-cell tolerogenic antigen presentation seems to be the dominant pathway in our model.

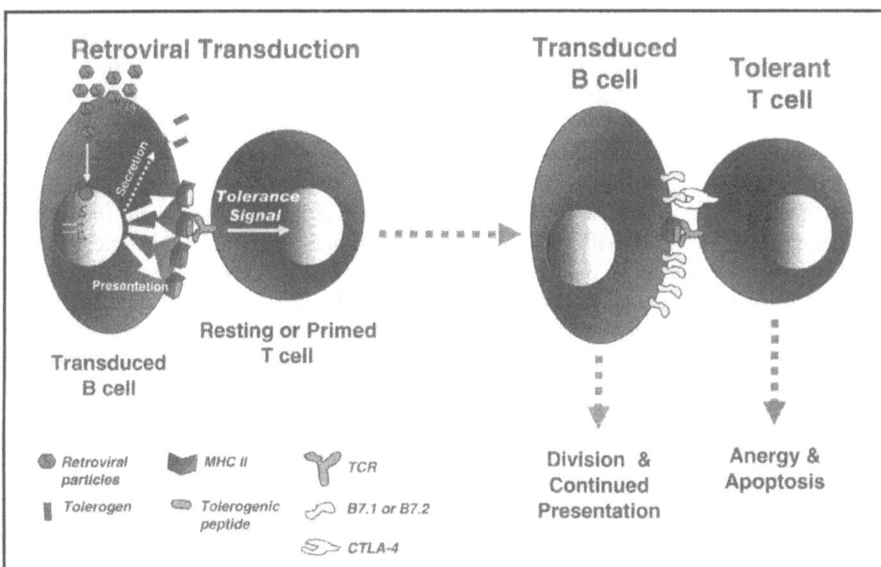

Figure 2. Mechanism of tolerance induction by an IgG-peptide.

Table 1. Expression of B7.2 by stimulated B cells in vivo

	Days				
	-2	**0**	**3**	**7**	**10**
LPS B	43.0	97.0	**77.5**	**67.5**	45.6
CpG B	43.0	94.2	**46.2**	**44.7**	36.3

Expression of B7.2 by Stimulated B Cells in vivo: Normal Balb/c recipients were injected with 5.5 x 106 CFSE-labeled, OVA-IgG B cells, stimulated for 48 hours in vitro with either LPS or CpG. Resting (day -2) and pre-injection (day 0) values of B7.2 expression were determined by flow cytometry. On days 3, 7, and 10, three animals were killed, and spleen cells were examined by flow cytometry to determine percentage of CFSE+ cells expressing B7. Values indicated in bold show a significant difference between groups.

Role of Co-Stimulation and the Mode of B-Cell Activation

Importantly, transfection of B cells requires their stimulation by mitogens in order to infect with retrovirus. In the past, we have used LPS and CD40L to stimulate our B cells with similar results. Since stimulation with LPS, e.g., upregulates B7.1 and B7.2 on B cells, this effectively eliminated lack of costimulation as a factor in the induction of tolerance by B cells. To examine the influence of different B-cell activators on IgG-peptide-induced tolerance, we stimulated BALB/c spleen cells with CD40L, CpG[21] oligonucleotides (active or inactive) or LPS. After 24hr, flow cytometry analysis of MHC class II and B220 expression showed a hierarchy of "activation" with CpG>CD40L>LPS (Fig. 3A). When these cells were then infected with retroviral vectors expressing the p12-26-IgG fusion proteins via our standard protocol, we found that both LPS and CD40L-activated B cells were tolerogenic, but that CpG activated B cells were not, in terms of proliferation (Fig. 3B), as well as IL-2 and IL-4 cytokine responses. We propose that this explains the utility of naked DNA vaccines for immunization because CpG sequences primed the mouse and acted as an adjuvant. Current data suggest that B7-family members are expressed on activated B cells at similar levels at 48 hrs; recent studies (Litzinger and Scott, in preparation, see Table 1) show that B7 expression is maintained for up to one week in vivo on LPS-activated B cells, but that these cells more quickly revert to a resting phenotype with CpG activation.

To further analyze the role of the B cell in this gene therapy protocol, retrovirally transduced B cells were labeled with carboxyfluorescein diacetate succinimidyl ester (CFSE) in order to track the proliferation, persistence, and phenotype of tolerogenic B cells in vivo, as well as to evaluate the effect of different stimuli on these tolerogenic B cells. We found that CFSE-labeled, retrovirally-transduced B cell blasts persisted in spleen for at least a month. By 7 days following transfer, more than 75 percent of the B-cell antigen-presenting cells have divided. The fate and phenotype of LPS vs. CpG stimulated transduced B cells are currently being further clarified.

We further tested the role of co-stimulation by treating recipients with anti-CTLA-4 to block the negative regulation by this receptor interacting with B7[22, 23] on the tolerogenic APC. Our results[20] suggest that blocking CTLA-4 interactions interferes with tolerance induction but only in primed hosts presumably because CTLA-4 is upregulated on primed but not naïve T cells;[23] in addition, anti-CTLA-4 may permit protective CD28:B7 interactions to occur. Since tolerance is relatively long-lived, this suggests that in vivo maintenance of tolerance probably occurs via a lack of co-stimulation but initially may require CTLA-4:B7 interactions based on the effects of anti-CTLA-4 treatment.

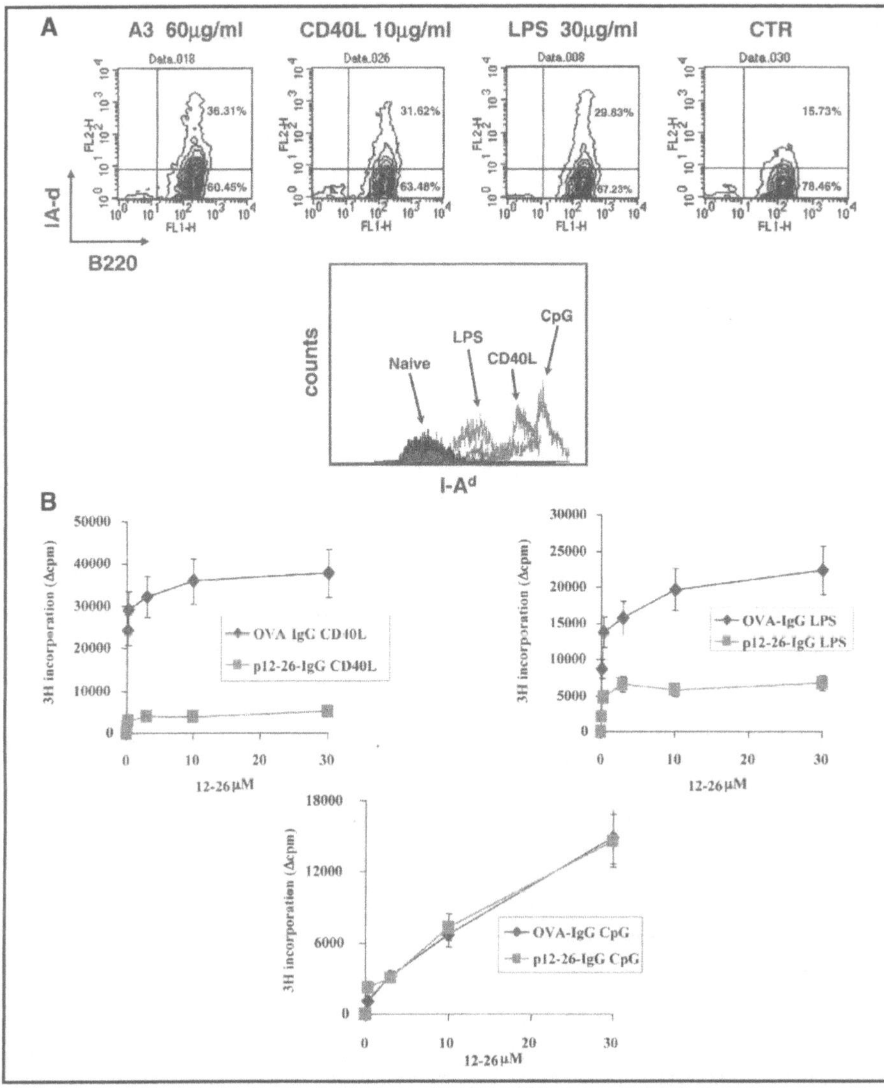

Figure 3. CpG oligomers promote survival and enhances activation of B cells. Splenocytes were stimulated for 24hrs with 30 µg/ml of LPS, 60 µg/ml of CpG (AT**CG**ACTCT**CG**AG**CG**TTCTC) and 10 µg/ml of CD40L. A) Cells were stained for B220 and I-A^d and analyzed on FACScalibur flow cytometer. B220$^+$ activated B cells with highest I-A^d surface expression are considered highly activated. Solid histogram represent unstimulated control; the remaining histograms are indicated by the arrows from left to right: LPS stimulated cells, CD40L stimulated cells; CpG stimulated cells. B) CpG activation of B cells modulates T cell tolerance induction. BALB/c mice were infused with 2x10^7 p12-26-IgG or OVA-IgG gene-transferred B cells from naive BALB/c mice stimulated for 24 hrs with CD40L (10 µg/ml), LPS (30 µg/ml) and CpG (60 µg/ml). Five days later, mice were immunized with 25 µg of p12-26 and 25 µg of OVA emulsified 1:1 in CFA. After immunization, lymph node T-cell proliferation (day 10-12) was measured against p12-26, the immunodominant epitope in H-2^d mice. Cultures were pulsed with [^{3}H] thymidine on day 3. One set of three representative experiments is shown, with pooled LN cells from 5 animals per group. Data are presented as mean cpm ± SE (Standard Error) above background, which was usually less than 1000-3000 cpm. OVA-IgG represents the control group retrovirally transduced with an unrelated construct, whereas p12-26-IgG represents experimental group.

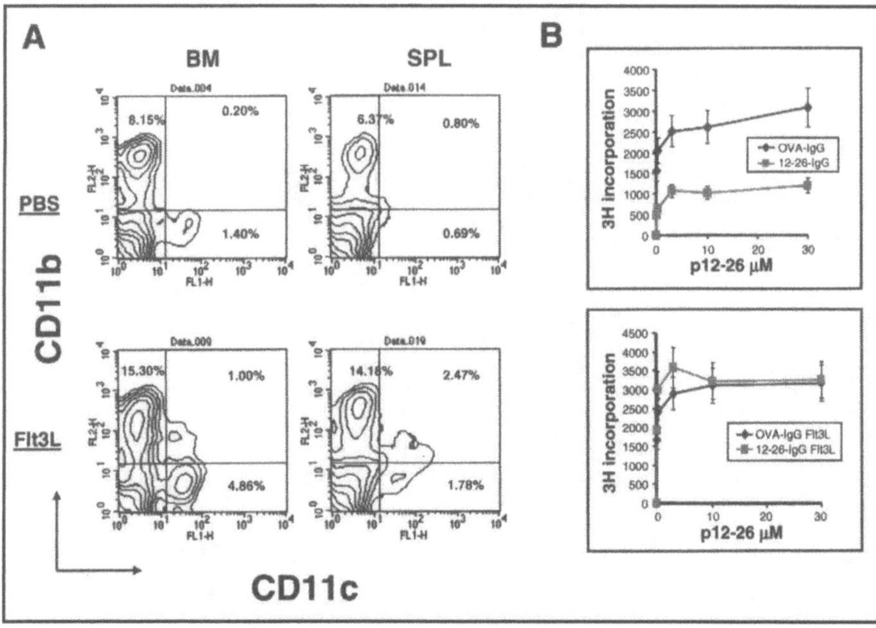

Figure 4. Recipients of retrovirally transduced bone marrow chimeras treated with Flt3L are not tolerant to p12-26. A) Spleen cells and Bone Marrow were stained for surface expression of CD11b and CD11c positive cells before and after injection with Flt3L. B) BALB/c mice were sub-lethally irradiated (300 Rad) and received 3 x 10^6 transduced BM cells intravenous (i.v.) and a week later received an injection of 10 µg/ml of hFlt3L (Immunex, Seattle, WA) or saline (control) daily for 10 days. Two weeks later, mice were immunized with 25 µg of p12-26 emulsified 1:1 with 25 µg of OVA in CFA. After immunization, lymph node T-cell proliferation (day 10-12) was measured against p12-26 the immunodominant epitope in H-2^d mice. Cultures were pulsed with [^{3}H] thymidine on day 3.

Knowing the importance of dendritic cells (DC) in immune tolerance and since the CpG treatment of B cells increases CD11c^+ cells we decided to investigate their role in our system. Therefore, we injected p12-26-IgG transduced BM cells into syngeneic irradiated recipients and then began a 10-day treatment with hFlt3L to enhance DC development. It's well known that Flt3L treatment induces the development of CD11c^+ / CD11b^+ DC,[24,25] which modulate different immune responses in different systems. Following the 10-day treatment, we observed both splenomegaly and an increase in CD11c, CD11b positive cells in bone marrow and spleen. Six weeks later when immune competence had been restored, BM chimeras were immunized and results showed that recipients of retrovirally transduced BM cells were not tolerant at the T-cell level when treated with Flt3L (Fig. 4). Presumably this is due to increased presentation by marrow-derived dendritic cells. While these data do not prove that DCs are immunogenic APCs in our system, it suggests that Flt3L treatment obviates the tolerogenicity of transduced B-cell precursors in the marrow. We still need directly test whether DC can be tolerogenic by transducing normal marrow cells and then differentiating them under DC or B-cell promoting conditions in vitro.

Recently, Zaghouani and co-workers[26] also reported that tolerance induced by peptide IgG conjugates may be optimized by aggregation of the IgG and the induction of IL-10 synthesis by activated T cells. While there are many differences between their system and ours (IgG2 vs. IgG1 carrier; neonatal vs. adult treatment; aggregated antigen is often immunogenic), the observation that IL10 is a powerful suppressor to TH1 responses led us to test a possible role of this cytokine in gene-transferred tolerance. Therefore, we used IL10 knockout (IL10-/-) mice as recipients of gene transferred bone marrow cells or bone marrow from IL10-/- or control mice. Our results show that IL-10 is not required for tolerance induction, nor is TH1/ TH2 skewing involved.[20]

In further experiments, in collaboration with Drs. Rajeev Agarwal and Rachel Caspi, we were unable to demonstrate a role for active suppression in gene-transferred tolerance since T-cells enriched from tolerant mice failed to transfer hyporesponsiveness.[27] However, these experiments need to be repeated, for example, with enrichment of CD25+ T cells with potential for suppressive activity, especially due to recent results in a diabetes model (see below).

Additional studies used *gld* B cells as a source of tolerogenic APC (in normal recipients which are not deficient in the Fas-FasL system). This was based on our finding that FasL was upregulated on LPS blasts. Our results initially suggested that cells lacking functional FasL (*gld*) were less effective as tolerogenic APC. While this result suggests the hypothesis that activation-induced cell death may be a major pathway of gene transferred tolerance, recent data from the Caspi lab demonstrated that *gld* B cells could be tolerogenic in a model of uveitis. Therefore, this area needs further investigation.

Applications for Clinical Models of Autoimmune Diseases

An important goal of our group has been to develop technology that can be applied for autoimmune diseases. As a first model, our lab collaborated with the Caspi lab at the National Eye Institute to examine this retroviral gene therapy approach for tolerance to an uveitogenic peptide (residues 161-180) from the interreceptor retinal binding protein[27] (IRBP). When this peptide coding sequence was inserted in frame in the IgG cassette and used as above, highly significant tolerance was achieved and dramatic diminution of disease was evident. This tolerogenic effect was stable for over six months! Importantly, with multiple injections of p161-180-IgG-transduced B-cell blasts, uveitis initiated by primed T cells could be reversed. More recent data also suggest that gene therapy with this immunodominant peptide construct could protect against challenge with the full-length IRBP protein (Caspi and Agarwal, personal communication).

In the EAE model, we engineered myelin basic protein (MBP)-IgG retroviral constructs to examine tolerance to encephalitogenic epitopes. Using a full-length MBP-IgG retroviral vector, we were able to reverse the transfer of EAE in different mice which have the potential to recognize different epitopes on MBP. Hence, to achieve clinical efficacy, one does not need to know the precise peptide sequences that bind to the appropriate MHC of the patient, unlike other procedures (such as specific peptide analogs), which require precise knowledge of the specific immunodominant class II epitope. Moreover, this protocol should work with different class II backgrounds, and other encephalitogenic proteins, like MOG and PLP, which is currently under study in the Scott lab. We have now extended these studies to treatment after disease symptoms have appeared (Melo and Scott, unpublished; see Fig. 5) and using B cells from MBP primed donors.

This system has now been extended to a spontaneous murine model for diabetes. Thus, we created full-length glutamic acid decarboxylase (GAD65)-IgG constructs and tested their efficacy in NOD mice, which spontaneously develop diabetes. In experiments, with a single treatment at 7-10 weeks (prior to overt clinical disease but with peri-insulitis) with this vector, we found a significant delay in the onset of diabetes, as measured by glucose levels and prolongation of life. In addition, a single treatment with either B cell transfected with GAD-IgG or with a second construct, insulin B9-23-IgG, after clinical signs of diabetes (week 14) showed less efficacy, although GAD was slightly better than the insulin B chain epitope.[28]

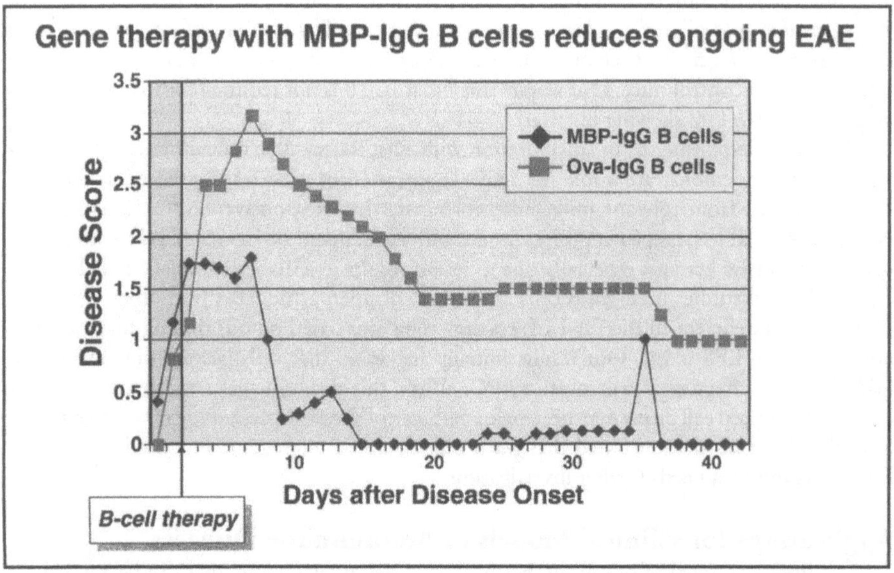

Figure 5. Effect of gene therapy with MBP-IgG retrovirally transduced primed B cells on ongoing EAE. Primed T cells from mice immunized with MBP in CFA were cultured with MBP + IL-2 and then used for passive transfer of disease to syngeneic recipients, which were boosted with MBP/CFA to increase disease incidence. Recipient mice were then monitored for EAE symptoms. Three days after disease onset, mice received primed B-cell blasts transduced with either a control construct (OVA-IgG) or the experimental construct (MBP-IgG); B cell donors were primed to mimic the situation in patients. Mice were distributed in each subgroup so that each group had the same number of sick animals and the same average score. Disease was monitored daily and average disease score calculated.

Because the islets are being destroyed by diabetogenic T cells once clinical symptoms appear, we wanted to test whether we could induce tolerance in primed T cells in animals with intact islets. Therefore, we transferred T cells from diabetic female mice to either NOD-scid (lacking an immune system) or NOD males, which have a low incidence of disease. We were unable to prevent diabetes in NOD-scid recipients, initially a disappointing result (Soukhareva and Scott, in preparation). However, complete prevention of the transfer of diabetes to male recipients occurred with GAD-IgG infected NOD B cells. These data show that clinical efficacy can be achieved with primed T cells and moreover that some host element, perhaps a regulatory T cell, might be involved in tolerance. Further studies in this system are in progress.

These results are highly encouraging as these not only provide proof of principle in several clinical disease models, but also support our hypothesis that large domains can be expressed in a tolerogenic manner for multiple epitopes contained therein.

References

1. Woods JM, Katschke KJ, Volin MV et al. IL-4 Adenoviral gene therapy reduces inflammation, proinflammation cytokines, vascularization, and bony destruction in rat adjuvant-induced arthritis. J Immunol 2001; 166:1214-1222
2. Chang Y, Prud'homme GJ. Intramuscular administration of expression plasmids encoding interferon-g receptor/IgG1 or IL-4/IgG1 chimeric proteins protects from autoimmunity. J Gene Med 1999; 1:415-423.
3. Costa GL, Sandora MR, Nakajima A et al. Adoptive Immunotherapy of experimental autoimmune encephalomyelitis via T cell delivery of the IL-12p40 subunit. J Immunol 2001; 167:2379-2387.

4. Takiguchi M, Murakami M, Nakagawa I et al. CTLA4-IgG gene delivery prevents autoantibody production and lupus nephritis in MRL/lpr mice. Life Sci 2000; 66:991-1001.
5. Quattrocchi E, Dallman MJ, Feldman M. Adenovirus-mediated gene transfer of CTLA4-Ig fusion protein in the suppression of experimental autoimmune arthritis. Arthritis Rheum 2000; 43:1688-1697.
6. Zambidis ET, Scott DW. Epitope-specific tolerance induction with an engineered immunoglobulin. Proc Natl Acad Sci USA 1996; 93:5019-5024.
7. Zambidis ET, Barth RK, Scott DW. Both resting and activated B lymphocytes expressing engineered peptide-Ig molecules serve as highly efficient tolerogenic vehicles in immunocompetent adult recipients. J Immunol 1997; 158:2174-2182.
8. Zambidis ET, Kurup A, Scott DW. Genetically transferred central and peripheral immune tolerance via retroviral-mediated expression of immunogenic epitopes in hematopoietic progenitors or peripheral B-lymphocytes. Mol Med 1997; 3:212-224.
9. Kang Y, Melo M, Deng E et al. Induction of hyporesponsiveness to intact foreign protein via retroviral-mediated gene expression: The IgG scaffold is important for induction and maintenance of immune hyporesponsiveness. Proc Natl Acad Sci USA 1999; 96:8609-8614.
10. El-Amine M, Melo M, Scott DW. Gene therapy for tolerance and autoimmunity: Soon to be fulfilled promises? Clin Immunol 2001; 99:1-6.
11. Melo M, El-Amine M, Tonnetti L et al. Gene therapeutic approaches to induction and maintenance of tolerance. Int Rev Immunol 2001; 20:627-645.
12. Scott DW, Venkataraman M, Jandinski JJ. Multiple pathways of B-cell tolerance. Immunol Rev 1979; 43:241-273.
13. Venkataraman M, Scott DW. Cellular events in tolerance. VII. Decrease in clonable precursors stimulatable in vitro by specific antigens or LPS. Cell Immunol 1979; 47:323-331.
14. Aldo-Benson M, Borel Y. The tolerant cell: direct evidence for receptor blockade. J Immunol 1974; 112:1793-1803.
15. Venkataraman M, Aldo-Benson M, Borel Y et al. Persistence of antigen-binding cells with surface tolerogen: Isologous versus heterologous immunoglobulin carriers. J Immunol 1977; 119:1006-1009.
16. Min B, Legge LK, Caprio JC et al. Differential control of neonatal tolerance by antigen dose versus extended exposure and adjuvant. Cell Immunol 2000; 200:45-55.
17. Kang J, Wither J, Hozumi N. Long-term expression of a T-cell receptor beta-chain gene in mice reconstituted with retrovirus-infected hematopoietic stem cells. Proc Natl Acad Sci USA 1990; 87:9803-9807.
18. El-Amine M, Hinshaw JA, Scott DW. In vivo induction of tolerance by an Ig peptide is not affected by the deletion of FcR or a mutated IgG Fc fragment. Int Immunol 2002; 14:761-766.
19. Ravetch JV, Bolland S. IgG Fc receptors. Ann Rev Immunol 2001; 19:275-290.
20. El-Amine M, Melo M, Kang Y et al. Mechanisms of tolerance induction by a gene-transferred peptide-IgG fusion protein expressed in B lineage cells. J Immunol 2000; 165:5631-5636.
21. Krieg AM, Yi AK, Matson S et al. CpG motifs in bacterial DNA trigger direct B-cell activation. Nature 1995; 374:546-549.
22. Bluestone JA. Is CTLA-4 a master switch for peripheral T cell tolerance? J Immunol 1997; 158:1989-1993.
23. Krummel MF, Allison JP. CD28 and CTLA-4 have opposing effects on the response of T cells to stimulation. J Exp Med 1995; 182:459-465.
24. Maraskovsky E, Brasel K, Teepe M et al. Dramatic increase in the numbers of functionally mature cells in Flt3 ligand-treated mice: Multiple dendritic cell subpopulations identified. J Exp Med 1996; 184:1953-1962.
25. Pulendran B, Smith JL, Jenkins M et al. Prevention of pripheral tolerance by a dendritic cell growth factor: Flt3 ligand as an adjuvant. J Exp Med 1998; 188:2075-2082.
26. Pack CD, Cestra AE, Min B et al. Neonatal exposure to antigen primes the immune system to develop responses in various lymphoid organs and promotes bystander regulation of diverse T cell specificities. J Immunol 2001; 167:4187-95.
27. Agarwal RK, Kang Y, Zambidis E et al. Retroviral gene transfer of an immunoglobulin-antigen fusion construct protects from experimental autoimmune uveitis. J Clin Invest 2000; 106:245-252.
28. Melo M, Qian J, El-Amine M et al. Gene transfer of Ig-fusion proteins into B cells prevents and treats autoimmune diseases. J Immunol 2002; 168:4788-4795.

Chapter 7

DNA Vaccination against Autoimmune Diseases

Gérald J. Prud'homme,* Yelena Glinka, Yigang Chang and Xiaoying Li

Introduction

The ultimate goal in the treatment of autoimmune diseases is to restore immune tolerance to the relevant target antigen(s). Short of this ideal, the attenuation of pathogenic immune responses is a highly desirable end. Many forms of immunotherapy are being studied with these objectives in mind, but gene transfer approaches, and particularly DNA vaccination (transfer of an antigen gene), are promising. DNA vaccination is most often performed by nonviral techniques, such as the intramuscular (i.m.) injection of naked plasmid DNA. In addition to antigen delivery, this approach permits local or systemic delivery of immunomodulatory molecules (DNA covaccination).[1-4] As reviewed below, DNA vaccination strategies have been employed to ameliorate autoimmune insulin-dependent diabetes mellitus (type 1 diabetes [T1D]), experimental autoimmune encephalomyelitis (EAE) and other autoimmune diseases.

An obvious limitation of systemic immunogene therapy involving delivery of cytokines, or other mediators, is that immune responses not relevant to a disease might be modified, possibly in a detrimental way. Toxic effects could also occur, if persistently elevated levels of circulating cytokines were generated. This is more likely to be a problem if vectors are readministered several times over a long period, as may be required in chronic diseases. On the other hand, DNA vaccination offers the possibility of modifying responses in an antigen-specific way after only a few DNA injections, which is a positive safety factor. In addition, DNA vaccination permits flexibility and options not otherwise possible. The inoculated plasmids can be easily modified, and immunomodulatory genes incorporated, to tailor immune responses in a very powerful way.

However, in terms of relevance to autoimmunity, DNA vaccines usually stimulate rather than depress immunity, primarily because plasmid DNA carries unmethylated CpG-containing immunostimulatory sequences (ISS).[5,6] It is now well established that these sequences bind to Toll-like receptor 9 (TLR9) expressed by dendritic cells (DCs) and some other cells, stimulating inflammatory cytokine production and initiating an innate immune response.[6] Thus, it has been challenging to construct DNA vaccines that suppress immunity in an antigen-specific way and, not surprisingly, both beneficial and detrimental effects have occurred. In this chapter, we discuss the features of protective vaccines, and the mechanisms that may be responsible for these positive effects.

*Gérald J. Prud'homme—Department of Laboratory Medicine and Pathobiology, St. Michael's Hospital, 30 Bond Street, Room 2013CC, Toronto, Ontario, Canada M5B1W8. Email: prudhommeg@smh.toronto.on.ca

Gene Therapy of Autoimmune Disease, edited by Gérald J. Prud'homme. ©2005 Eurekah.com and Kluwer Academic / Plenum Publishers.

DNA Vaccination

DNA vaccines stimulate humoral, T-helper (Th) and cytotoxic T lymphocyte (CTL) responses against encoded antigens (reviewed in refs. 4, 7-14) usually of infectious agents or tumors, and can be delivered by i.m. (most studied), intradermal/epidermal, subcutaneous, or mucosal routes. As discussed further below, immunity can be enhanced by coinjecting cytokine plasmids (or bicistronic plasmids), and can be biased to a Th type 1 (Th1) or Th type 2 (Th2) type.

Antigen Uptake and Presentation

Studies with bone marrow chimeras reveal that after delivery (i.m. or other) of an antigen-encoding vector the expressed antigens are presented by bone marrow-derived or "professional" antigen presenting cells (APCs),[15] presumably DCs. It is still unclear how APCs acquire antigen, but two mechanisms are plausible. There could be direct transfection of APCs by plasmid, or uptake of protein from other transfected cells (cross presentation). Cross presentation can lead to enhanced immunity (cross priming) or depressed immunity (cross tolerance).

Both mechanisms of antigen uptake appear to occur, and their relative importance is still under study. Ablation of muscles a few minutes after DNA injection does not prevent immunization,[16] which is difficult to explain if myocytes are the sole producers of antigen. Indeed, following i.m. injection, plasmids can be identified in draining lymph nodes and many other tissues, and transfection could be occurring in these sites. Moreover, some reports suggest direct transfection of DCs.[17-18] Despite these findings, strong evidence of cross-presentation comes from the finding that transplantation of myoblasts transfected to express influenza NP protein induces both antibodies and CTLs against that antigen.[19-20] In addition, a study[21] suggests that though direct transfection of DCs occurs, the bulk of the immune response is dependent on antigen expression by nonlymphoid tissues and transfer to APCs. In accord with this, it proved possible to induce strong immunity against a hepatitis B envelope protein by DNA vaccination with a plasmid carrying a muscle-specific desmin promoter,[22] where antigen production was presumably limited to myocytes. Also mitigating against direct presentation, the uptake of DNA by mononuclear cells is associated with extensive DNA degradation and low or undetectable reporter protein synthesis.[23]

In muscle, antigen will be expressed longer than in most other tissues, which could explain, at least in part, why the i.m. route has been superior in several DNA vaccination studies. Interestingly, in vivo electroporation markedly enhances the effectiveness of DNA vaccination,[23,24] perhaps due to increased transfection of either muscle cells, other nonlymphoid cells, or APCs. Indeed, the local delivery of multiple long squarewave electric pulses (20-30 msec) of low voltage (50-200 V/cm) shortly after the administration of naked DNA in various tissues improves transfection efficiency by 10-1000 fold.[23-30] Furthermore, as an additional mechanism, mild muscle damage as may be induced by electroporation could provoke an influx of APCs, as well as release of antigen from injured cells, thereby increasing antigen presentation.

CpG Motifs and TLR9

An important component of the plasmid is the presence of unmethylated CpG-containing immunostimulatory sequences (ISS), that can activate innate immunity by binding to TLR9.[5,6,31] The features of these CpG motifs are described in Chapter 3 (Piccirillo et al), and are only briefly discussed here. Engagement of TLR9 triggers a cell signaling cascade involving myeloid differentiation primary response gene 88 (MyD88), and several other elements, resulting in the activation of NFκB. Cells that express TLR9, which include plasmacytoid dendritic cells (PDCs) and B cells, produce interferon α and β (IFNα/β), inflammatory cytokines such as IL-12, and chemokines.

Optimal CpG motifs for activating mouse or rabbit immune cells have the general formula, purine-purine-CG-pyrimidine-pyrimidine. However, for activating human cells, and cells of several other species, the optimal motif is TCGTT and/or TCGTA. In addition, some sequences that are immediately adjacent to these short motifs can contribute to the immunostimulatory effects. Three classes of CpG-containing oligodeoxynucleotides (ODNs) have been described.[31] CpG ODNs of the B-class (also called K-class) strongly stimulate B cells, promote PDC maturation, but induce only low amounts of IFNα/β. In contrast, A-class (also called D-class) ODNs strongly stimulate plasmacytoid DCs (PDCs) to secrete IFNα/β, but are poor at activating B cells. C-Class ODNs combine the properties of the A and B classes, and are very strong Th1 adjuvants. The high levels of IFNα induced by either A-class or C-class ODNs activate NK cells efficiently. Moreover, CpG ODNs promote the transition from monocytes to myeloid DCs, and contribute to DC maturation. Interestingly, mice lacking TLR9 can still respond to DNA vaccination,[32] indicating that there are other pathways of immune activation, yet to be described.

It is important to note that some CpG ODNs do not stimulate, but rather inhibit responses, although the mechanisms of suppression are not well understood. Suppressive motifs are rich in polyG or -GC sequences, tend to be methylated, and are present in the DNA of mammals and certain viruses.[32] These neutralizing motifs (CpG-N motifs) also exit in plasmids. Most DNA vaccines contain numerous CpG motifs, some of which are in an immunostimulatory context, while others are inhibitory. Thus, the ultimate effect of the plasmid DNA backbone in DNA vaccination may depend on the ratio of stimulatory and inhibitory sequences. In DNA vaccination against autoimmune diseases, the contribution of the stimulatory versus inhibitory CpG motifs carried by vectors has not been extensively studied, and this is an obvious area for future investigation. It is noteworthy, however, that CpG ODNs can induce the production of regulatory cytokines such IL-10 and TGF-β1,[33-35] which have many direct immunoinhibitory effects, and can promote the differentiation of some types of regulatory T cells (see Chapter 3). Furthermore, Moseman et al.[36] observed that human plasmacytoid DCs activated by CpG ODNs induce the generation of $CD4^+CD25^+$ regulatory T (Tr) cells. These Tr cells express forkhead transcription factor 3 (Foxp3) and produce IL-10, TGF-β, IFNγ, and IL-6, but low IL-2 and IL-4. These studies suggest there are various mechanism by which CpG motifs can suppress immunity. It remains unclear, however, under which circumstances ODNs will favor immunity versus suppression.

Regulation of Th1, Th2 and CTL Activity by DNA Vaccination

In mice, immunity can be enhanced by coinjecting cytokine expression plasmids (or use of bicistronic plasmids), and can readily be biased to a Th1 or Th2 type as shown by several investigators in various models (Table 1).[4,7-11,37-39] For example, we found that i.m. injections of a plasmid encoding carcinoembryonic antigen (CEA) elicited both humoral and cellular immune responses, but only delayed the growth of transplanted syngeneic CEA^+ tumor cells.[38,39] Coinjection of the CEA vector with a vector encoding either IFNγ or IL-12 (bicistronic p35/p40) promoted a Th1 response, anti-CEA CTL activity and resulted in up to 80% tumor-free survival following a challenge. In contrast, coinjection of the CEA vector with an IL-4 vector produced a Th2 response, and a reduction in CTL activity. Resistance to a tumor challenge was also decreased.

Many cytokines are effective costimulatory adjuvants, boosting humoral as well as Th- and CTL-mediated responses (Table 1). Moreover, coinjection of B7-1, B7-2 and CD40L

Table 1. Examples of cytokine gene effects in DNA vaccination

Gene	Humoral Immunity	Th1-Type Response	Th2-Type Response	CTL
GM-CSF	↑[a]	↑	↑	↑
IFNγ	— or ↑ or ↓	↑	↓	↑
TGF-β1	↓	↓	— or ↑	?
IL-1	↑	↑	↓	↑
IL-2	↑	↑	— or ↑ or ↓	↑
IL-4	↑	↓	↑	↓
IL-8, IP-10, or MIP-1alpha	↑	↑	—	—
IL-10	↑	↑or ↓	↑	—
IL-12	↑ or—	↑	↓	↑

a. ↑, increased; ↓, decreased; —, unchanged. In almost all cases, the antigen and cytokine genes were codelivered as either a two-plasmid mixture or a bicistronic plasmid. Injection of the antigen and cytokine plasmids at separate sites, or at the same site separated in time, is frequently ineffective. Some responses have differed between studies, possibly for technical reasons. In addition, most studies were conducted in rodents by i.m. injection, and responses may vary depending on the mode of delivery and between species. Reviewed or reported in references 4, 7-11, 37-39.

genes, on the same or separate plasmid(s) as the antigen gene, can markedly improve the effectiveness of DNA vaccines.[10] It is important to note, however, that the results outlined in Table 1 have been obtained mostly in mice and might not applicable to all species. In cattle, for example, DNA vaccination skews responses almost exclusively to a Th2 type.[40] In fact, a number of studies using T cell clones suggest that the classical roles of many cytokines in the mouse do not extrapolate entirely or at all to cattle.[40] In humans, experience with strictly plasmid-based DNA covaccination is very limited. The majority of DNA vaccination clinical trials have been performed with "prime-boost" strategies incorporating cytokine-encoding viral vectors, and this approach is considerably different from most DNA covaccination studies in mice.

DNA Vaccination and Immune Tolerance

DNA vaccination can break tolerance to self or transgenic "neo-self" antigens. Notably, Davis et al[41] induced immune responses against HBsAg in HBsAg transgenic mice. The induction of autoimmunity by DNA vaccination has been most clearly demonstrated in tumor models. Amici et al,[42] found that i.m. injections of plasmids encoding segments of the rat neu (erbB2) oncogene in FVB neu-transgenic (neu^+ mammary cancer-prone) mice induced anti-neu immunity and exerted an anti-tumor effect. Coinjection of an IL-12 plasmid improved the response.

Almost all tumor-associated antigens (TAAs) in humans are normal, nonmutated self molecules. Thus, the induction of any immune response to these antigens involves breaking natural immune tolerance, and might result in autoimmunity. As an example, melanocyte differentiation antigens are potential target TAAs for specific melanoma immunotherapy. To override tolerance, xenogeneic DNA immunization has been exploited. Small differences in the expressed xenoprotein sequence often results in immune recognition of self-molecules. For instance, immunizing mice with DNA coding for the xenogeneic human melanosomal membrane glycoprotein gp100 overcomes tolerance and results in tumor immunity.[43] In this case, class I major histocompatibility complex (MHC) molecules are required, and the immunized mice demonstrate autoimmunity manifested as coat color depigmentation (vitiligo). This type of response is improved by coupling DNA vaccination with electroporation.

Similarly, immunity to tyrosinase-related protein-1 (TRP-1) expressed by melanocytes has been investigated in a mouse model.[44] C57BL/6 mice generated antibodies against mouse TRP-1 after DNA immunization against human TRP-1. Immunization against the mouse molecule did not have this effect. Acquired immunity to TRP-1provided significant anti-tumor protection, but autoimmunity was observed in the form of coat depigmentation. Interestingly, protection from a melanoma tumor challenge required $CD4^+$ and $NK1.1^+$ cells and the Fc receptor γ-chain, but depigmentation was independent of these components. Thus, DNA immunization broke tolerance against a mouse TAA, possibly by providing help from $CD4^+$ T cells. The mechanisms required for resisting a tumor challenge were different from those causing autoimmunity, suggesting that these two phenomena can be uncoupled.

DNA vaccination has been exploited as a means of inducing organ-specific autoimmunity in animals. A transgenic mouse expressing lymphocytic choriomeningitis virus nucleoprotein (NP) under the control of a liver-specific promoter developed liver injury when vaccinated with plasmids expressing NP as an intracellular or a secretory protein.[45] Coinjection of an IL-12 bicistronic plasmid that we constructed[39] with an NP plasmid facilitated the induction of a Th1 phenotype. CTLs activated in peripheral lymphoid organs by DNA vaccination migrated to the periportal and lobular areas of the liver. Their presence was associated with a significant degree of cytolysis, as evidenced by elevated transaminases several weeks after immunization.

Autoimmunity has also been induced against the thyroid gland in outbred NMRI mice, by vaccination with a plasmid encoding the human thyrotropin receptor (TSHr).[46] The mice produced antibodies reactive to TSHr, and some showed signs of hyperthyroidism including elevated total T4 and suppressed TSH levels. The mice developed goiters with extensive lymphocytic infiltration, and displayed ocular signs similar to those of Graves' disease. Thus, this creates a remarkably convincing murine model of Graves' disease.

It is of some concern that transfected muscle cells may be attacked and injured by the immune system following DNA vaccination against foreign antigens, and indeed this has been reported (reviewed in refs. 9, 10). A related concern is the production of pathogenic anti-DNA antibodies, potentially induced by plasmid DNA and its ISS motifs. This risk appears small, but nevertheless exists,[31] as discussed further in Chapter 3. Though modest increases in anti-DNA titers have been reported in DNA-vaccinated normal mice, these antibodies are usually reactive to hypomethylated bacterial DNA or ssDNA from mammalian sources, but not mammalian dsDNA. This presumably results from sequence motifs that differ between bacterial and mammalian DNA and can be recognized as foreign. These antibodies are not usually pathogenic.[10,31] In lupus-prone mice, anti-dsDNA antibodies titers may be increased by DNA vaccination, presumably due to polyclonal activation of pre-existing self-reactive B cells and, for reasons that are not fully elucidated, the severity of disease may be either increased, not altered or even reduced.[10,31,47,48]

Table 2. Alteration of EAE by DNA vaccination

Species	Vaccine (cDNA)	Covaccine (cDNA)	Disease Severity[a]	Postulated Mechanism of Protection	Refs.
mouse	TCR-Vβ8.2	none	↓	Th2 bias	49
mouse	TCR-Vβ8.2	none	↓	Tr, IFNγ↑	50
mouse	PLP139-151	none	↓	Anergy	54
mouse	PLP139-151	IL-4	↓	Th2 bias	59
	MOG	IL-4	↓	Th2 bias	59
mouse	PLP139-151	none	↑		55
mouse	MOG	none	↑		56
rat	MBP68-85	AACGTT (CpG)	↓	T-cell response↓	58
	MBP68-85	IL-4	↑		58
rat	MBP68-85	Protein A analogue	↓	IFNγ↓	62
rat	MOG91-108	Protein A analogue	↑		51
rat	MIP-1α, MCP-1, or FasL	none	↓	Immunity to encoded cytokine or FasL	63, 64

a. ↑, increased; ↓, decreased.

EAE

Despite reports of autoimmunity induction, under some circumstances DNA vaccination against either autoantigens, T-cell receptor (TCR) variable elements, or even inflammatory cytokines, has depressed immunity. EAE (Table 2) and T1D are the diseases for which DNA vaccination has been most extensively tested. An early report [49] relied on inducing immunity to a TCR element. A variable region gene of the TCR, Vβ8.2, is rearranged, and its product is expressed on pathogenic T cells that cause EAE in $H\text{-}2^u$ mice after immunization with MBP. Vaccination of these mice with naked DNA encoding Vβ8.2 protected mice from EAE. Analysis of T cells reacting to the pathogenic portion of the MBP molecule indicated that in the vaccinated mice there was a reduction in the Th1 cytokines IL-2 and IFNγ, combined with an elevation of IL-4, a Th2 cytokine believed to protect against disease.

More recently, the induction and involvement of regulatory T-cell (Tr) responses has been investigated in a similar model.[50] Using mutant Vβ8 DNA molecules and cell transfer strategies, it was demonstrated that Tr cells are involved in mediating skewing of the anti-MBP response in a protective Th2 direction and prevention of disease. Vaccination of B10.PL mice with plasmid DNA encoding the TCR Vβ8.2 gene segment resulted in significant protection from EAE. The protection was specific in that vaccination with DNA encoding the TCR Vβ3 gene segment, not displayed on disease-causing T cells, did not influence the course of disease. Furthermore, the Vβ8.2 DNA-mediated protection involved CD4 T cells reactive with the dominant determinant from the FR3 region of the Vβ8.2 chain. Vaccination with mutant Vβ8.2 DNA encoding point mutations in the FR3 region, critical for recognition by T cells, did not prevent EAE, whereas vaccination with mutant Vβ8.2 DNA encoding alterations in an irrelevant region of the TCR chain was protective. Prevention of EAE was accompanied by deviation of the anti-MBP Ac1–20 (the target peptide) response in a Th2 direction. Surprisingly, however, the $CD4^+$ Tr cells involved in this process secrete IFNγ, an inflammatory cytokine that usually suppresses Th2 responses, and their mechanism of action is unclear.

These results should be interpreted with some caution because IFNγ has protective effects in EAE that are not apparent in multiple sclerosis (MS), T1D, lupus and some other autoimmune diseases.[51] Notably, while IFNγ neutralization or depletion protects against T1D and lupus, it is detrimental in EAE.[52,53] Another caveat is that the autoaggressive T-cell repertoire in EAE is much more restricted than in natural autoimmune diseases such as T1D in nonobese diabetic (NOD) mice. Thus, TCR variable elements are unlikely to be ideal targets in many autoimmune diseases.

A simpler and more direct approach to disease prevention involves DNA vaccination against the target autoantigen. In this case, tolerance induction is clearly linked to antigen recognition, and may or may not influence other immune responses depending on the mechanism of action. This approach is counterintuitive since DNA vaccines generally enhance responses, and could aggravate disease. Indeed, studies of DNA vaccination against autoantigens in EAE have shown both positive and negative effects, sometimes with very similar protocols of immunization. Some authors reported protection against EAE by vaccination with DNA encoding a minigene for residues 139-151 of myelin proteolipid protein (PLP139-151), a pathogenic self antigen.[54] Previously DNA-vaccinated SJL/J mice were protected against the induction of disease by administration of encephalitogenic peptide emulsified in CFA. Proliferative responses and production of the Th1 cytokines, IL-2 and IFNγ, were reduced in T cells responsive to PLP139-151. In the brains of mice that were successfully vaccinated, mRNA for IL-2, IL-15, and IFNγ were reduced. The authors suggested that tolerance was induced through T-cell anergy. However, another group[55] obtained conflicting results with plasmids encoding whole PLP or encephalitogenic epitopes PLP139-151 and PLP178-191. DNA vaccination with these plasmids enhanced R-EAE initiated by immunization with peptides or whole PLP in adjuvant. Thus, DNA vaccination was detrimental, and the reasons for discrepancies with the previously described study are unclear.

Other investigators[56] also observed negative effects in a related model of EAE. They assessed the potential of vaccination with a DNA construct encoding the myelin oligodendrocyte glycoprotein (MOG). Mice vaccinated with MOG-DNA developed an exacerbated form of EAE when challenged with either MOG or the unrelated encephalitogen PLP. DNA vaccination failed to tolerize the MOG-specific T-cell response and led to the concomitant induction of a cytopathic MOG-specific autoantibody response, which was pathogenic, enhancing demyelination, inflammation and disease severity. This model differs from classical MBP-induced models in that antibodies appear to be pathogenic. In most other types of EAE pathology has been attributed to Th1 cells. These differences in pathogenesis should be taken into account when interpreting the results of vaccination studies.

There is evidence that the timing of DNA vaccination relative to disease induction (or sensitization) is very important. Thus, in one study[57] early sensitization for EAE (4 weeks after DNA vaccination) caused recipient mice to develop an exacerbated form of disease, while late sensitization (>10 weeks) resulted in an ameliorated form. In the mice sensitized early post-DNA vaccination, a Th1-type response was noted. In contrast, late sensitization led to peripheral tolerance as evidenced by a decrease in T-cell proliferation and CTL response, without a Th2 response.

The presence of CpG DNA has an influence on the outcome of anti-EAE DNA vaccination. On the basis that ISS in the plasmid backbone are necessary for efficient DNA vaccination, some authors[58] have studied the effect of one such ISS, the 5'-AACGTT-3' motif. Treatment with a DNA vaccine encoding MBP68-85 and containing three ISS of 5'-AACGTT-3' sequence suppressed clinical signs of EAE, while a corresponding DNA vaccine without such ISS had no effect. There was reduced proliferative T-cell responses in rats treated with the

ISS-containing DNA vaccine, compared with controls. Coinjection of IL-4-, IL-10-, or TNFα-coding cDNA inhibited the suppressive effect of the DNA vaccine on EAE, whereas GM-CSF-coding cDNA had no effect. Coinjection of cytokine-coding cDNA with the ISS-deficient DNA vaccine failed to alter clinical signs of EAE. It is unclear, however, how ISS influenced the response in a positive way. Since most plasmids contain numerous CpG motifs, that may be either stimulatory or inhibitory, it is always difficult to analyze CpG-related effects.

From these studies it is evident that, at least in EAE-related diseases, DNA vaccination against a target antigen yields unpredictable results. Clinically, this approach against autoimmunity should only be considered with great caution. However, there is evidence that vaccines can be modified such that they are more reliably protective. One approach is to include a regulatory cytokine gene. Garren et al[59] demonstrated that codelivery of the IL-4 gene and a DNA vaccine encoding PLP139-151 induced protective immunity against EAE. They also showed that DNA vaccines can be used to reverse established MOG35-55-induced EAE by covaccination with cDNA for MOG and IL-4. Unlike vaccination without IL-4, which induced anergy, the introduction of IL-4 rescued T cells from anergy and promoted differentiation to a Th2 phenotype.

Unfortunately, these results may not be applicable to other species. For example, addition of an IL-4 gene had a negative effect on DNA vaccination in a rat model of EAE,[58] and Th2 deviation was detrimental in a primate model of EAE.[60] These results highlight the risks of modifying responses with cytokines. Most of these mediators have pleiotropic effects and can have stimulatory or inhibitory effects depending on the concentration, target cells or tissue, and interactions with other cytokines in the milieu. Furthermore, the pathogenic mechanisms of autoimmunity are complex and can vary markedly from one species to another. Another caveat is that protective effects can be highly antigen specific. Notably, a single amino acid exchange in position 79 from serine (nonself) to threonine (self) in MBP dramatically altered the protection against rat EAE.[61] Vaccines encoding the encephalitogenic sequence MBP68-85 did not protect against the second encephalitogenic sequence MBP89-101 in Lewis rats and vice versa. To these limitations, we must add that induced diseases such as EAE are undoubtedly much simpler than natural diseases, where there is often autoreactivity to multiple antigenic determinants and autoantigens, presumably due to the occurrence of widespread intra- and intermolecular determinant spreading during the course of disease.

Another potential approach to improving vaccines involves linking the antigen to immune-related ligands. For instance, Lobell et al[62] vaccinated Lewis rats with DNA encoding an encephalitogenic T-cell epitope, guinea pig MBP peptide 68-85 (MBP68-85), before induction of EAE with MBP68-85 in complete Freund's adjuvant (CFA). They fused the antigenic peptide to a protein A analogue that binds to Fc of IgG. Compared to vaccination with a control DNA construct, the vaccination suppressed clinical and histopathological signs of EAE, and reduced the IFNγ production after challenge with MBP68-85. They report that targeting of the gene product to Fc of IgG is essential for this effect, and protection is not related to a Th2 cytokine bias. The mechanisms of protection, however, remain to be elucidated and the in vivo effects of the protein A construct are likely to be diverse.

Moreover, these results were not applicable to another model of EAE. MOG91-108 is encephalitogenic in DA rats and MHC-congenic LEW.1AV1 ($RT1^{av1}$) and LEW.1N ($RT1^{n}$) rats.[51] DNA vaccination with a tandem MOG91-108 construct suppressed MOG peptide-induced EAE, and all investigated rat strains were protected. However, there was no requirement for targeting the gene product to IgG. Surprisingly, in complete contrast to the previous study, MOG peptide fusion with a protein A analogue abolished the protective effect of the vaccine. Th1-promoting CpG DNA motifs in the plasmid backbone of the construct were necessary for efficient DNA vaccination. The authors failed to detect any effects on ex vivo MOG-peptide-induced IFNγ, TNFα, IL-6, IL-4, IL-10, and brain-derived neurotropic factor expression in splenocytes or CNS-derived lymphocytes. MOG-specific IgG2b responses were enhanced after DNA vaccination. The enhanced IgG2b responses together with the requirement for CpG DNA motifs in the vaccine suggest a protective mechanism involving induction of a Th1-biased immune response.

In view of the conflicting results obtained in different models of EAE, it is difficult at present to judge the usefulness of targeting autoantigen to Fc with protein A analogues. It is also unclear if this method has similar effects to those obtained by directly fusing the antigen to IgG-Fc, which is a method discussed later in this chapter.

Some authors have designed protective DNA vaccines by targeting cytokines or chemokines.[63,64] They report that plasmid-inoculated animals develop antibodies or other immune responses against these mediators. Plasmids encoding different C-C chemokines were administered in vivo. Induced immune responses to macrophage-inflammatory protein-1α (MIP-1α) or monocyte-chemotactic protein-1 (MCP-1) prevented EAE. It appears that suppression of EAE with C-C chemokine DNA vaccines is dependent on targeting chemokines that are highly expressed in the CNS at the onset of disease. Similarly, administration of a FasL plasmid[65] broke tolerance and elicited immunity to FasL. FasL-specific autoantibodies isolated from immunized rats inhibited the in vitro production of TNFα by cultured T cells, and were protective when administered to rats at the onset of EAE, but detrimental when delivered later.

Interestingly, DNA vaccination against osteopontin, an inflammatory cytokine believed to play a role in the pathogenesis of EAE and MS, induces anti-osteopontin antibodies and ameliorates MOG35-55-induced EAE (L. Steinman and colleagues, text in www.sciencemag.org/cgi/reprint/299/5614/1845b).

In these cases it has been proposed that there is autoreactivity to the immune mediator encoded by the plasmid. This is surprising since these mediators are self molecules that are ubiquitously expressed in practically all immune responses and/or inflammatory reactions. It is surprising that DNA vaccines that activate innate immunity through their ISS sequences could induce this type of autoimmunity which has not, to our knowledge, been reported following DNA immunization against pathogens or tumors. In any case, these phenomena should be investigated thoroughly, as autoimmunity against cytokines could have long-lasting and unpredictable effects. It should also be considered that the cytokine plasmids might have acted, at least in part, by modifying the immune response irrespective of autoimmunity against the encoded product.

Autoimmune Diabetes

Antigenic Targets in NOD Mice

NOD mice develop an autoimmune form a diabetes (T1D), more severe in females, where insulin-producing β cells are destroyed following infiltration of islets of Langerhans by macrophages and islet-cell antigen reactive, autoaggressive T cells.[66-69] The islet inflammatory process is termed insulitis. The disease can be adoptively transferred with T lymphocytes, provided both $CD4^+$ and $CD8^+$ cells are included, and diabetogenic T-cell clones reactive to various islet antigens have been isolated. The development of diabetes is greatly accelerated by administering cyclophosphamide (CYP), which induces a burst of IFNγ production for reasons that have not been elucidated.

DNA vaccination is essentially a form of antigen therapy, and it is critically important to choose the correct target antigen. However, in some spontaneous autoimmune diseases the relevant target antigen(s) are either unknown or, as in the case of T1D, several have been identified. Thus, the development of antigen-based therapies has involved considerable trial and error. Antigen therapy for protection against diabetes, most often with protein antigens, has been extensively reviewed,[70-79] and due to space limitations can only be briefly discussed.

Some protective methods of vaccination, such as administration of complete Freund's adjuvant (CFA) or BCG do not target a specific antigen,[80-82] while others are directed at TCR determinants.[83,84] Application of these techniques in humans is problematic, or not possible. For instance, CFA cannot be used due to its inflammatory/necrotizing effects and BCG does not seem effective.[72,85] Targeting the TCR is limited by variable TCR usage in autoaggressive clones and, furthermore, anti-TCR immunity sometimes aggravates autoimmune disease.

Several islet-cell antigens have been recognized: proinsulin/insulin, glutamic acid decarboxylase isoforms 65 and 67 (GAD65, GAD67), IA-2 and related tyrosine phosphatases, p69, heat shock protein 60 (HSP60), carboxypeptidase H, gangliosides and others (reviewed in Refs. 72-78). GAD isoforms and insulin are the best studied, but the relative importance of the various islet antigens has not been clear. In humans, GAD65 is a well-established target autoantigen in Stiff Man syndrome (SMS; a neurological disease), and two out of three of these patients also have T1D[70] suggesting an association. In NOD mice anti-GAD immunity occurs early,[86] and a study showed that β-cell specific suppression of GAD65/67 expression in antisense GAD transgenic mice prevents insulitis and diabetes.[87] Protective unresponsiveness to GAD, or protective Th2 bias, have been induced in some studies.[72,74-78] Somewhat surprisingly, transgenic expression of GAD65 in multiple tissues does not tolerize NOD mice,[88] though expression limited to islets sometimes does. NOD mice with GAD65 gene knockout still develop diabetes[90] and, clearly, other antigens are being targeted.

Tian et al[86] propose that a Th1 biased autoimmune response against GAD occurs spontaneously, concurrent with the onset of insulitis. Subsequently, the response spreads intramolecularly and intermolecularly (determinant spreading). Tisch et al[91] report that induction of GAD65-specific Th2 cells and suppression of IDDM at late stages of disease is epitope dependent. Paradoxically, NOD IL-4 null mice do not have a more severe disease,[92] Th2 clones are not protective in cotransfer experiments,[93,94] and they can induce disease in NOD.scid mice.[94] Perhaps protection is mediated by nonTh2 regulatory T cells (Tr).[2] Indeed, T cells of NOD mice expressing a transgenic TCR reactive to a GAD65 peptide did not induce diabetes, but rather had a protective effect in adoptive transfer experiments.[95]

Insulin is an autoantigen in T1D in humans and NOD mice[77] and, thus far, has shown the greatest potential for antigen therapy. Administration of insulin, or its B:9-23 peptide, to NOD mice either orally, nasally, or i.v. protects from diabetes,[80,96-100] possibly by biasing responses to a Th2 type, or inducing other Tr cells.[96-98] A study by Delovitch and colleagues[101] reveals that a peptide spanning the B-C junction of proinsulin I (p24-33 epitope) is an early autoantigen epitope in the pathogenesis of type 1 diabetes. Very early immunization against this peptide was protective, but immunization initiated at 5 wk of age was detrimental. Wegmann et al[102] found that T cells reactive to insulin B:9-23 form a large part of the islet-infiltrating population in NOD mice, and others[103-105] have reported pathogenic CTLs reactive to the same epitope. Insulin B-chain reactive clones have been isolated from diabetic patients.[78]

The diabetes prevention trial (DPT-1), where insulin was administered s.c. and i.v. to individuals at risk of developing diabetes, has yielded negative results.[77] Part of the trial involving oral administration of insulin was also unsuccessful. However, though oral tolerance induction is an attractive possibility, it has been difficult to reliably induce this type of tolerance in humans.[72,74,106] These negative results are consistent with our own negative findings with DNA vaccination against unmodified preproinsulin (PPIns; see below), as well as the observations of others[101] that tolerance induction with proinsulin peptides can be highly age restricted. Nevertheless, we observed protection from diabetes in NOD mice after coinoculation of plasmids encoding the protease furin and mutated preproinsulin cleavable by furin (FIns) (unpublished). This allows production of mature insulin by muscle cells. Our results in NOD mice suggest that either FIns is more tolerogenic or that the protective effect is nonimmunological but dependent on the production of active insulin, and we are investigating this question.

Table 3. Alteration of autoimmune diabetes by DNA vaccination

Diabetes Model	Vaccine (cDNA)	Covaccine (cDNA)	Disease Severity	Postulated Mechanism of Protection	Refs.
TG RIP-LCMV[b]	Ins B	none	↓[a]	Th2 bias	109
TG	PPIns, PIns, Ins	none	↑		110
RIP-B7.1[c]	GAD65	none	—		110
NOD	Empty	none	↓	Th2 bias	107
	HSP60	none	↓	Th2 bias	107
NOD/CYP	HSP60	none	↓	Th2 bias	108
NOD	Ins B9-23	none	↓	IFNγ↓	111
NOD	Ins B9-23	none or IL-4	↓	Th2 bias	112
NOD	InsA-IgG-Fc	none or IL-4	—		113
	InsB-IgG-Fc	none or IL-4	↑		113
NOD	PPIns	none	—		151
	PPIns	B7-1wa (CTLA-4 ligand)	↓	T-cell anergy	151
NOD	GAD65	none	—		114
NOD	GAD65	none	↓		115
NOD	rVV-GAD65	none	↓	Th2 bias	116
NOD	GAD65	none	—		117
	spGAD (secreted)	none	↓	IL-10↑, TGFβ1↑	117
NOD/CYP	GAD55 (secreted)	none	↓	Th2 bias	121
NOD	GAD65-IgG-Fc[d]	none	—		113, 135
	GAD65-IgG-Fc[d]	IL-4	↓	Th2 bias	113, 135

a. ↑, increased; ↓, decreased; —, unchanged.
b. TG RIP-LCMV, transgenic mice with islet-restricted expression of lymphocytic choriomeningitis virus nucleoprotein under the control of the rat insulin promoter (RIP).
c. TG RIP-B7, transgenic mice with islet-restricted expression of B7.1 under the control of the rat insulin promoter (RIP).
d. GAD65-IgG-Fc, GAD65-segment construct fused to an IgG-Fc segment.

Plasmid Inoculation in NOD Mice

Several DNA vaccination approaches have been protective in diabetes-prone mice (Table 3). We have not observed any protective effects following i.m. injection of empty plasmid vectors in NOD mice, and most other authors report similar findings. However, Quintana et al[107] found that NOD diabetes could be inhibited by vaccination with either a pcDNA3 empty vector, a DNA construct encoding human heat shock protein 60 (HSP60), or an oligonucleotide containing a CpG motif. Prevention of diabetes was associated with a decrease in the degree of insulitis and with down-regulation of spontaneous proliferative T-cell responses to HSP60 and its peptide p277. Both the pcDNA3 vector and the CpG oligonucleotide induced specific antibodies primarily of the IgG2b isotype to HSP60 and p277, and not to other islet antigens (GAD or insulin) or to an unrelated recombinant antigen expressed in bacteria. Protection with empty plasmid may depend on the specific plasmid backbone, or other poorly understood factors, and was not observed in CYP-accelerated diabetes.[108]

Almost all other studies have shown a requirement for antigen. In one study, vaccination with pHSP60[108] modulated the T cell responses to HSP60 and also to the GAD and insulin autoantigens. T-cell proliferative responses were significantly reduced, and the pattern of cytokine secretion to HSP60, GAD, and insulin was characterized by an increase in IL-10 and IL-5 secretion and a decrease in IFNγ secretion, compatible with a shift from a Th1 to a Th2 response.

In other DNA vaccination studies, as summarized below, the antigens targeted have included insulin (either preprosinsulin, proinsulin, B-chain, or A-chain), GAD isoforms, GAD-derived peptides and some antigen-Ig fusion constructs. In addition, transgenic models of diabetes have been investigated.

DNA Vaccination against Insulin

Coon et al[109] used mice expressing lymphocytic choriomeningitis virus nucleoprotein (LCMV-NP) as a transgene in their beta cells. These mice develop insulin-dependent diabetes mellitus only after LCMV infection. Inoculation of plasmid DNA encoding the insulin B chain reduces the incidence of IDDM by 50% in this model. DNA vaccination induces regulatory CD4 lymphocytes that react with the insulin B chain, secrete IL-4, and locally reduce activity of LCMV-NP-autoreactive CTLs in the pancreatic draining lymph node. This disease, however, could differ significantly from the spontaneous disease of NOD mice. Moreover, insulin is not always protective in transgenic models. Karges et al[110] observed that i.m. insulin DNA vaccination can initiate autoimmune diabetes in two mouse models of type 1 diabetes. This was the case in NOD mice immunized with PPIns DNA. In contrast, GAD65 DNA conferred protection, and empty vector was ineffective. In RIP-B7.1 C57BL/6 mice (expressing the immune costimulatory molecule B7.1 in pancreatic beta-cells), autoimmune diabetes occurred in 70% of animals after PPIns vaccination, but not after GAD65 or control DNA administration. When induced, diabetes was characterized by $CD4^+$ and $CD8^+$ T-cell infiltration of islets of Langerhans and severe insulin deficiency. Interestingly, PPIns, proinsulin, and insulin DNA were equally effective for disease induction. However, in our studies we did not find that immunization against PPIns or GAD65 (unmutated) significantly altered the incidence of diabetes in NOD mice, although modest effects were apparent in some experiments. These differences between studies could be related to the different vectors and/or methods used.

In any case, DNA immunization against insulin constructs has often either not changed the incidence of disease or has increased it. Vaccination against the insulin B-chain only has yielded mixed results. Urbanek-Ruiz et al[111] immunized NOD mice with a plasmid encoding residues 9-23 of the B chain. Animals injected i.m. had a lower disease incidence and delayed onset of disease. Surprisingly, in this study, proliferative responses to insulin and other islet cells antigens were not altered and insulitis was not diminished. The reasons for the favorable outcome are unclear. There was, however, decreased production of IFNγ by pancreatic lymph nodes in response to insulin, suggesting immune deviation. Similarly, Bot et al[112] found that expression of insulin B chain initiated early in life by plasmid inoculation resulted in the protection of female NOD mice against disease. This was associated with a Th2 shift in spleen, expansion of IL-4-producing and, to a lesser extent, of IFNγ-secreting T cells in pancreatic lymph nodes, as well as intermolecular Th2 epitope spreading to GAD determinants. IL-4-null NOD mice still developed diabetes, implying a role for this cytokine. Male NOD mice did not respond favorably to insulin B DNA vaccination, but this was corrected by adding an IL-4-expressing plasmid or extension of the vaccination schedule.

Contrasting results were obtained by Weaver et al[113] who examined the immunotherapeutic efficacy of plasmid DNA encoding murine insulin A and B chains fused to IgG-Fc. Administration of the insulin B-chain construct, with or without IL-4, precipitated the onset of insulitis and diabetes. This correlated with increased number of IFNγ-producing $CD4^+$ and

$CD8^+$ T cells in response to insulin B chain peptide stimulation. Treatment with plasmid DNA encoding insulin A chain-IgG-Fc had no effect on disease. However, covaccination with GAD65-IgG-Fc and IL-4 cDNA prevented IDDM. This study and others confirm that insulin- and GAD65-specific T-cell reactivity induced by DNA vaccination have distinct effects on the progression of IDDM. The role of the IgG segment in this study is unclear, although other studies have suggested that it has a positive effect on tolerance induction, possibly because it is secreted and enters the circulation, binds to immunoinhibitory Fc receptors, and/or alters antigen uptake and presentation by APCs.

DNA Vaccination against GAD65

Like in the case of insulin, DNA vaccination against GAD65 in NOD mice has yielded some contradictory results. The first published study[114] showed no effect on disease incidence, although anti-GAD antibodies were identified. However, it was later reported that DNA vaccination against GAD65 reduced the incidence of diabetes, and moderately ameliorated insulitis, although T-cell responses to this antigen were not markedly altered and regulatory T cells were not generated.[115] B7/CD28 costimulation with bicistronic GAD65/B7 plasmids abrogated the beneficial effect. Protective effects have also been reported in a GAD65 vaccinia viral-vectored (rVV-GAD65) model.[116]

Administration of rVV-GAD65 to NOD mice prevented diabetes in an age-dependent and dose-dependent manner. The anti-GAD response was shifted to a Th2 type and, furthermore, splenocytes from rVV-GAD65-treated NOD mice prevented the adoptive transfer of diabetes in NOD.scid recipients.

In contrast to these studies, we found that i.m. DNA vaccination against wild-type GAD65 (full length protein) was not protective in NOD mice.[117] Surprisingly, there was little evidence that the procedure was modifying T-cell immunity to GAD65. This protein is cytosolic and it lacks a signal for the secretory pathway. We hypothesized that it might not be efficiently picked up and presented by antigen presenting cells (APCs). We constructed an expression plasmid encoding a chimeric GAD65-derived molecule (spGAD) with a signal peptide originating from IL-4, a secretable protein, to facilitate the release of this antigen. This protein was secreted in culture, albeit not efficiently, following transient transfection of COS-7 cells with the plasmid vector (denoted VR-spGAD). In contrast to the unmodified GAD65 vector, immunization with VR-spGAD had a protective effect against diabetes, which was apparent in mice receiving multiple injections of the plasmid. This was accompanied by reduced insulitis scores, indicating that there was an anti-inflammatory effect at the level of the islets.

Moreover, VR-spGAD induced alterations in the response of lymphocytes. We observed increased secretion of both IL-10 and IFNγ in response to GAD65 peptide stimulation in vitro, and a decrease in the IFNγ/IL-10 ratio in culture supernatants, compared to mice immunized with a blank plasmid or one encoding GAD65. Similarly, VR-spGAD-immunized mice had high serum IL-10 levels and low serum IFNγ levels compared to other groups, suggesting a systemic effect. Spontaneous in vitro production of TGF-β1 by the spleen cells of nondiabetic mice, but not diabetic animals, was observed and production of this cytokine was enhanced by antigenic stimulation with either GAD65 peptides or insulin.

These alterations in regulatory cytokine production were apparent both early and late after the treatment was initiated, and persisted for months after the last of multiple DNA injections. There was no notable change in the production of IL-4 in any of the groups, perhaps reflecting the reduced ability of NOD mice to produce this cytokine. Taken together, these alterations do not suggest a classical Th1 to Th2 switch in the response. It appears more likely that DNA vaccination with VR-spGAD protects NOD mice by increasing regulatory cytokine production (IL-10 and TGF-β1). This cytokine production pattern corresponds most closely to the Tr1 type of regulatory T cell,[73,118-120] and this question should be investigated further. Interestingly, another group has reported that DNA vaccination to a secreted form of GAD (GAD55) is protective in CYP-treated NOD mice[121] suggesting that this approach is applicable to both spontaneous and drug-induced disease.

A similar cytokine secretion pattern was reported recently in GAD65 T-cell receptor (TCR) transgenic mice.[122] These mice did not develop diabetes and their T cells protected NOD mice against diabetes in adoptive cotransfer experiments. The T cells of these animals proliferated in response to a GAD65 peptide and secreted IL-10, IFNγ, IL-2 and TNFα. We speculate that our method of DNA vaccination could be generating this type of regulatory T cell. Interestingly, $CD4^+CD25^+$ regulatory T cells, that are thought to act by direct cell contact rather than secretion of cytokines, may act by inducing other cells to produce IL-10 or TGF-β.[123,124] They could also be implicated in the protection associated with spGAD vaccination.

A notable feature of vaccination against VR-spGAD was a reduction in the serum levels of IFNγ. This is in accord with our previous observations that the neutralization of IFNγ by gene therapy with its soluble receptor reduces the incidence of diabetes in NOD mice.[125,126] Moreover, the alterations in the serum IFNγ/IL-10 ratio we are reporting are similar to the observations of another group.[127] It seems increasingly likely that the ratio of these two cytokines is a relevant factor, perhaps more important than the exact level of each cytokine. IL-10 has many immunosuppressive and anti-inflammatory effects that could block autoimmunity.[124] Indeed, IL-10 reduces MHC and B7-2 expression on APCs, induces T-cell anergy, promotes the differentiation of regulatory T cells, and increases T-cell apoptosis.[124,128] Others have reported that systemic delivery of IL-10,[129] IL-10-Ig fusion protein,[130] or IL-10-producing islet-reactive T-cell clones[131] protects NOD mice against diabetes. Taken together, these results suggest that disease is likely to progress when mice have a high IFNγ/IL-10 ratio, but not when they have a low ratio. Thus, successful immunotherapies and/or vaccines should aim to produce a low ratio. Based on our findings, increased TGF-β1 production could also be an important factor. Indeed, we reported that delivery of this cytokine by intramuscular gene transfer prevents diabetes in NOD mice.[132]

The Level of Antigen Expression in Tissues

There is evidence that the level of antigen expression in tissues affects the outcome of DNA vaccination. In a RIP-LCMV virally induced type 1 diabetes model, the endogenous expression levels of GAD determined whether DNA immunization with this antigen was beneficial or detrimental.[133] The authors analyzed the effect of vaccination with GAD65 plasmids in mice expressing high or low levels of GAD in their β islet cells. Lower expression levels in β cells supported induction of regulatory Th2-like cells, and protected from disease. Higher levels of islet GAD favored Th1-like autoaggressive responses and aggravation of disease. Coimmunization with an IL-4-expressing plasmid reduced the risk of augmenting autoaggression and in this way increased the safety margin of this immune-based therapy.

The level of antigen expression after DNA vaccination in inoculated tissues might also be an important factor. However, there is very little published quantitative data on the level of antigen produced in DNA vaccination studies. The work of Hartikka et al[134] demonstrated that alterations in plasmid constructs could alter reporter protein production in muscle by over 100 fold. It seems likely that antigen expression in the experiments described in this chapter could have varied by at least that much from one study to another. In our studies, we used the backbone elements of a plasmid described by Hartikka et al,[134] VR1255 (Vical Inc., San Diego, CA), that promotes very high expression in muscle. This vector has CMV immediate-early enhancer-promoter elements, CMV intron A, and a rabbit β-globin transcriptional terminator. Moreover, we have frequently added in vivo electroporation which, as mentioned above, also greatly enhances expression. Therefore, our results are based mostly on high antigen expression experiments, which might account for differences with other studies. We have also found that cytokine genes can rapidly shut down vector expression, while nonimmune genes are often expressed for periods of months. Thus, GAD65 protein was produced in muscles for months after an injection of GAD65 plasmid.[117] The persistence of antigen production is likely to be an important factor for tolerance induction. Evidently, many variables affect DNA vaccination and their full significance has not been determined.

Modification of the Antigen by Fusion with IgG-Fc

Tisch et al[135] constructed plasmids encoding a secreted fusion protein consisting of a fragment of GAD65 linked to IgG-Fc. The GAD65 fragment contained three peptide epitopes (amino acid residues 206–220, 217–236, and 290–309), which are recognized by $CD4^+$ T-cell clones derived from unimmunized or GAD65-immunized NOD mice. I.m. injection of plasmid DNA coexpressing GAD65-IgG-Fc and IL-4 protected NOD mice from diabetes, whether they were treated at early or late preclinical stages of disease. The protection reported by Tisch et al[135] was antigen-specific, inasmuch as plasmid DNA encoding hen egg lysozyme-IgG-Fc and IL-4 was ineffective. This beneficial effect appears related to GAD65-specific regulatory Th2 cells, which are induced by the addition of IL-4 cDNA. It can be presumed that IL-4 negates, at least in part, the Th1-inducing effects of ISS carried by plasmid. We have observed a similar effect when vaccinating against a tumor antigen.[38]

Consistent with a beneficial effect of IL-4, Tisch et al[135] found that GAD65-specific Th1 cell reactivity was significantly enhanced in animals immunized with plasmid DNA encoding GAD65-IgG-Fc without IL-4. They also observed that IL-4-null mice were not protected by their DNA vaccine, confirming an important role for this cytokine. A notable feature in these experiments is that vaccination begun at 12 weeks of age, when NOD mice already have insulitis, reduced the incidence of diabetes markedly. Thus, the vaccine does not have to be administered before the onset of autoimmunity to be effective.

Notably, vaccination against unmodified GAD65, with or without IL-4, was not successful,[135] suggesting that the IgG-Fc segment plays an important part in tolerance induction. It seems plausible, in view of other results with secreted GAD, that secretion of the IgG-Fc construct is a key feature, but the Fc segment could also be acting by other mechanisms as mentioned previously.

Immunoinhibitory DNA Vaccines

The negative regulator CTLA-4 is another potential target for immunotherapy. This molecule is expressed following activation of T cells, and its mode of action is complex and incompletely understood (see refs. 136,137 for recent reviews). CTLA-4 is underexpressed in NOD mice[138] and in humans, some polymorphisms of the gene increase susceptibility to insulin-dependent diabetes mellitus (IDDM) and other autoimmune diseases.[139,140] CTLA-4 blockade with monoclonal antibodies (mAbs) provokes autoimmunity in TCR transgenic and normal mice.[141-143] Moreover, CTLA-4 is expressed by a population of regulatory $CD4^+CD25^+$ T cells (5-10% of peripheral $CD4^+$ cells) that is thought to protect against autoimmunity. Spontaneous diabetes is exacerbated in B7-1/B7-2-deficient or CD28-deficient NOD mice, and these mice have a profound decrease in $CD4^+CD25^+$ regulatory T cells.[144] Interestingly, treatment of NOD mice with CD3 mAb boosts the activity of these regulatory T cells.[73] It has been proposed that these regulatory cells act by direct contact and independently of either CTLA-4 or soluble mediators.[119,120] However, Read et al[145] report that the suppressive activity of these (or similar) Tr cells in vivo depends on the expression of CTLA-4 and production of TGF-β1. This is consistent with reports[146-148] that cross-linking of CTLA-4 induces production of TGF-β1 by T cells.

Taken together, these findings suggest that increasing negative signaling could prevent autoimmunity, and that CTLA-4 is a potential target. CTLA-4, like CD28, binds B7-1/2[136,137] and its use has been limited by the lack of a selective natural ligand. It is possible to specifically engage CTLA-4 with mAbs, but antibody therapy usually masks CTLA-4 and boosts immune responses.[136] To avoid these limitations, we designed plasmids encoding a mutant form of B7-1 (W88>A; denoted B7-1wa) that binds CTLA-4 but not CD28.[149,150] We found that i.m. codelivery of a B7-1wa plasmid blocked DNA immunization as hypothesized.[151]

In NOD mice, delivery of either PPIns or B7-1wa cDNA alone did not suppress the autoimmune anti-insulin response of spleen cells.[151] However, codelivery of B7-1wa and PPIns cDNA (amplified by in vivo electroporation) abrogated reactivity to insulin and ameliorated disease. IFNγ and IL-4 were both depressed, arguing against a Th2 bias. Reactivity to GAD65 peptides was not reduced, suggesting that the induction of tolerance was restricted to insulin. Cell mixing experiments revealed that the spleen cells of insulin-tolerant mice could not suppress the anti-insulin response of spleen cells of naive NOD mice. Protection against diabetes was partial (50-60% reduced incidence) in these experiments. It appears that tolerance was induced by either T-cell anergy or deletion. The reduction in disease incidence was improved to 75% when PPIns was replaced by a PPIns-GAD65 fusion gene (Ins-GAD; unpublished). In this case, the proliferative response of spleen cells in response to both GAD65 peptides and insulin was reduced. However, IL-10 and TGF-β1 production was enhanced in response to GAD65 peptides or insulin. Moreover, vaccination generated regulatory T cells that protected NOD.*scid* mice in adoptive transfer experiments (manuscript in preparation).

We hypothesize that IL-10 production is initiated by a response against GAD65 rather than against insulin (we did not see this effect when immunizing with PPIns + B7-1wa). Ins-GAD, like spGAD, is found in both the cell lysates and culture supernatants of transfected COS-7 cells (unpublished observation). Therefore, it shares features with spGAD, but also carries insulin antigenic determinants. We postulate that Ins-GAD will be a superior vaccine due to the induction of tolerance against a large number of target epitopes, and/or generation of regulatory T cells. A key questions is whether human molecules similar in properties to mouse B7-1wa can be generated. The work of Fargeas et al[152] reveals that an equivalent mutation in human B7-1 (W84>A) abrogates binding to CD28 but not CTLA-4. Thus, it appears feasible to generate human DNA vaccines that would target CTLA-4 by our method. Furthermore, T cells express other immunoinhibitory molecules (e.g., PD-1) that might be targeted with similar effect.

DNA Vaccination against Arthritis

The feasibility of vaccination with naked DNA encoding for mycobacterial heat shock protein 65 (HSP65) in the modulation of experimental arthritis has been studied. In the model of adjuvant arthritis (AA) rats inoculated with CFA, which contains killed mycobacteria, develop an arthritis where HSP65 is thought to be an important target antigen. AA was induced in Lewis rats preimmunized i.m. with a plasmid encoding for HSP65.[153] The HSP65 plasmid-treated treated rats were significantly protected from disease development in comparison with the control groups. This finding correlated with the results of histologic and radiologic examinations of the involved joints. T-cell proliferation and antibodies to this protein were found to be elevated in treated rats when compared with both the arthritic control (adjuvant-induced) and the naive (did not receive adjuvant) animals. The mechanism of protection has not been elucidated.

As in EAE, vaccination against chemokines has also been found to be beneficial.[154] Administered naked DNA vaccines encoding MIP-1α, MCP-1, MIP-1β and RANTES to Lewis rats revealed that each of these vaccines induced immunity to the corresponding gene product. Upon induction of AA, this immunity appears to have contributed to the inhibition of disease. Self-specific anti-chemokine antibodies developed in DNA-vaccinated animals and were neutralizing in vitro These antibodies could adoptively transfer the beneficial effect of each vaccine. Remarkably, repeated administration of the constructs encoding MCP-1, MIP-1α, or RANTES inhibited the development and progression of AA, even when each vaccine was administered only after the onset of disease. In a similar study,[155] the administration of a TNFα DNA construct after the onset of disease led to a rapid, long-lasting remission.

DNA Vaccination against Carditis

DNA vaccination has been employed to rapidly vaccinate against pathogenic TCR elements, and this was most notably demonstrated in a rat carditis model.[156] Experimental autoimmune carditis-associated TCRs, Vβ8.2 and Vβ10, were determined by complementarity-determining region 3 (CDR3)-spectratyping analysis and subsequent sequencing of the relevant CDR3 regions. DNA vaccination against both Vβ8.2 and Vβ10 TCRs ameliorated autoimmune carditis and completely abrogated inflammation in some animals.

DNA Vacination against Lupus

DNA vaccination against lupus seems poorly indicated in view of the anti-DNA autoimmunity characteristic of this disease. Nevertheless, some interventions are feasible.

Fan and Singh[157] identified MHC class I-binding epitopes in the heavy chain variable region of anti-DNA antibodies from lupus-prone (NZB/NZW F1) mice. DNA vaccination to these epitopes induced $CD8^+$ T cells that killed anti-DNA antibody-producing B cells, reduced serum anti-DNA antibody levels, ameliorated nephritis and improved survival.

Concluding Remarks and Future Prospects

DNA vaccination against autoimmune diseases is a new approach that has shown both promise and limitations. There has been rapid progress in understanding how CpG motifs affect the immune response, and this may facilitate future development. Stimulatory elements can be depleted in favor of inhibitory elements, and this approach is being investigated. Overall, the results reviewed in this chapter do not suggest that classical DNA vaccination against an autoantigen will predictably protect against autoimmunity. On the contrary, it appears that detrimental effects are just as common as beneficial ones. This comes as no surprise, since DNA vaccines are generally immunostimulatory. It has been unclear which vector elements or factors determined a favorable outcome. This has led investigator to test vaccines that incorporate genes encoding immunomodulatory elements, particularly cytokines. This approach has produced positive results, and might lead to safer vaccines. However, there are significant interspecies differences in the response to these vaccines, and clinical studies must be conducted with caution. Other molecules, such as B7-1wa that binds to CTLA-4, act on immunoinhibitory molecules and appear to have more specific suppressive effects on the immune response. If similar ligands can be designed for human studies, then antigen-specific and safe immunoinhibitory vaccines are likely to be produced.

There are many variables that need to be further studied. This includes considerations such as antigen modification (e.g., secretion and construction of Ig fusion products), the level and length of vector expression, the effects of electroporation when it is applied, the choice of target tissues and the method of DNA delivery. The role of various DC subpopulations must also be established with greater precision, and this is another area where rapid progress is being made. ISS can induce DCs to produce both IL-10 and IL-12,[158,159] and we speculate that some protective effects are related to the secretion of IL-10. Perhaps ISS sequences can be fashioned to favor the production of regulatory cytokines. In any case, the introduction of regulatory cytokine genes into DNA vaccines is a simple alternative which should be more extensively studied. On the other hand, CpG-mediated stimulation of DCs can induce the production of IL-6 which has recently been found to antagonize the activity of $CD4^+CD25^+$ Tr cells.[160] This type of cytokine-dependent interaction is obviously detrimental to vaccination against autoimmune diseases. DNA vaccines might be improved if IL-6 or other cytokines that negatively affect regulatory T cells were somehow neutralized.

There are important differences in the response of human and mouse DCs to CpG elements that will undoubtedly affect the response to DNA vaccines. Another consideration is that transfection efficiency, at least in muscle, is lower in large mammals than in rodents, and methods of DNA delivery will have to be adapted accordingly. Nevertheless, several recent studies reveal that DNA vaccination is feasible in humans, dogs, pigs, and other large species. These studies are almost all designed to test immunostimulatory vaccines, but there are no obvious reasons to believe that inhibitory vaccines cannot be produced. Thus far, DNA vaccines have had an impressive safety profile. Indeed, there are good reasons to be optimistic about the future in this area. A major advantage of DNA vaccines over other immunotherapeutic methods is their remarkable simplicity. This approach is straightforward and inexpensive, and when it is sufficiently developed could be easily applied in the clinic by any physician.

Acknowledgements

Our studies were funded by the Juvenile Diabetes Foundation International, the Canadian Diabetes Association and the National Cancer Institute of Canada. We thank Vical Inc. for providing the VR1255 plasmid utilized in our studies.

References

1. Prud'homme GJ. Gene therapy of autoimmune diseases with vectors encoding regulatory cytokines or inflammatory cytokine inhibitors. J Gene Med 2000; 2:222-232.
2. Prud'homme GJ, Piccirillo CA. The inhibitory effects of transforming growth factor beta-1 (TGF-β1) in autoimmune diseases. J Autoimmunity 2000; 14:23-42.
3. Garren H, Steinman L. DNA vaccination in the treatment of autoimmune diseases. Curr Dir Autoimmun 2000; 2:203-216.
4. Scheerlinck JY. Genetic adjuvants for DNA vaccines. Vaccine 2001; 19:2647-2656.
5. Krieg AM. Antitumor applications of stimulating toll-like receptor 9 with CpG oligodeoxynucleotides. Curr Oncol Rep 2004; 6:88-95.
6. Krieg AM. CpG motifs in bacterial DNA and their immune effects. Annu Rev Immunol 2002; 20:709-60.
7. Prud'homme GJ, Lawson BR, Chang Y et al. Immunotherapeutic gene transfer into muscle. Trends Immunol 2001; 22:149-155.
8. Cohen AD, Boyer JD, Weiner DB. Modulating the immune response to genetic immunization. FASEB J 1998; 12:1611-1626.
9. Donnelly JJ, Ulmer JB, Shiver JW et al. DNA vaccines. Annu Rev Immunol 1997; 15:617-648.
10. Gurunathan S, Klinman DM, Seder RA. DNA vaccines: Immunology, application, and optimization. Annu Rev Immunol 2000; 18:927-974.
11. Gurunathan S, Wu CY, Freidag BL et al. DNA vaccines: A key for inducing long-term cellular immunity. Curr Opin Immunol 2000; 12:442-447.
12. Payne LG, Fuller DH, Haynes JR. Particle-mediated DNA vaccination of mice, monkeys and men: Looking beyond the dogma. Curr Opin Mol Ther 2002; 4:459-466.
13. Dunham SP. The application of nucleic acid vaccines in veterinary medicine. Res Vet Sci 2002; 73:9-16.
14. Muthumani K, Kudchodkar S, Zhang D et al. Issues for improving multiplasmid DNA vaccines for HIV-1. Vaccine 2002; 20:1999-2003.
15. Iwasaki A, Torres CA, Ohashi PS et al. The dominant role of bone marrow-derived cells in CTL induction following plasmid DNA immunization at different sites. J Immunol 1997; 159:11-14.
16. Torres CA, Iwasaki A, Barber BH et al. Differential dependence on target site tissue for gene gun and intramuscular DNA immunization. J Immunol 1997; 158:4529-4532.

17. Casares S, Inaba K, Brumeanu TD et al. Antigen presentation by dendritic cells after immunization with DNA encoding a MHC class II-restricted viral epitope. J Exp Med 1997; 186:1481-1486.
18. Chattergoon MA, Robinson TM, Boyer JD et al. Specific immune induction following DNA-based immunization through in vivo transfection and activation of macrophages/antigen-presenting cells. J Immunol 1998; 160:5707-5718.
19. Ulmer JB, Deck RR, Dewitt CM et al. Generation of MHC class I-restricted cytotoxic T lymphocytes by expression of a viral protein in muscle cells: Antigen presentation by nonmuscle cells. Immunology 1996; 89:59-67.
20. Fu TM, Ulmer JB, Caulfield MJ et al. Priming of cytotoxic T lymphocytes by DNA vaccines: Requirement for professional antigen presenting cells and evidence for antigen transfer from myocytes. Mol Med 1997; 3:362-371.
21. Corr M, von Damm A, Lee Dj et al. In vivo priming by DNA injection occurs predominantly by antigen transfer. J Immunol 1999; 163:4721-4727.
22. Kwissa M, von Kampen K, Zurbriggen R et al. Efficient vaccination by intradermal or intramuscular inoculation of plasmid DNA expressing hepatitis B surface antigen under desmin promoter/enhancer control. Vaccine 2000; 18:2337-2344.
23. Dupuis M, Denis-Mize K, Woo C et al. Distribution of DNA vaccines determines their immunogenicity after intramuscular injection in mice. J Immunol 2000; 165:2850-2858.
24. Widera G, Austin M, Rabussay D et al. Increased DNA vaccine delivery and immunogenicity by electroporation in vivo. J Immunol 2000; 164:4635-4640.
25. Tamura T, Sakata T. Application of in vivo electroporation to cancer gene therapy. Curr Gene Ther 2003; 3:59-64.
26. Zhang L, Nolan E, Kreitschitz S et al. Enhanced delivery of naked DNA to the skin by noninvasive in vivo electroporation. Biochim Biophys Acta 2002; 1572:1-9.
27. Li S, Benninger M. Applications of muscle electroporation gene therapy. Curr Gene Ther 2002; 2:101-105.
28. Somiari S, Glasspool-Malone J, Drabick JJ et al. Theory and in vivo application of electroporative gene delivery. Mol Ther 2000; 2:178-187.
29. Mathiesen I. Electropermeabilization of skeletal muscle enhances gene transfer in vivo. Gene Ther 1999; 6:508-514.
30. Mir LM, Bureau MF, Gehl J et al. High-efficiency gene transfer into skeletal muscle mediated by electric pulses. Proc Natl Acad Sci USA 1999; 96:4262-4267.
31. Klinman DM. Immunotherapeutic uses of CpG oligodeoxynucleotides. Nat Rev Immunol 2004; 4:249-58.
32. Spies B, Hochrein H, Vabulas M et al. Vaccination with plasmid DNA activates dendritic cells via Toll-like receptor 9 (TLR9) but functions in TLR9-deficient mice. J Immunol 2003; 171:5908-5912.
33. Jain VV, Kitagaki K, Businga T et al. CpG-oligodeoxynucleotides inhibit airway remodeling in a murine model of chronic asthma. J Allergy Clin Immunol 2002; 110:867-872.
34. Yi AK, Yoon JG, Yeo SJ et al. Role of mitogen-activated protein kinases in CpG DNA-mediated IL-10 and IL-12 production: central role of extracellular signal-regulated kinase in the negative feedback loop of the CpG DNA-mediated Th1 response. J Immunol 2002; 168:4711-4720.
35. Lammers KM, Brigidi P, Vitali B et al. Immunomodulatory effects of probiotic bacteria DNA: IL-1 and IL-10 response in human peripheral blood mononuclear cells. FEMS Immunol Med Microbiol 2003; 38:165-172.
36. Moseman EA, Liang X, Dawson AJ et al. Human plasmacytoid dendritic cells activated by CpG oligodeoxynucleotides induce the generation of $CD4^{+}CD25^{+}$ regulatory T cells. J Immunol 2004; 173:4433-4442.
37. Kim JJ, Trivedi NN, Nottingham LK et al. Modulation of amplitude and direction of in vivo immune responses by coadministration of cytokine gene expression cassettes with DNA immunogens. Eur J Immunol 1998; 28:1089-103.
38. Song K, Chang Y, Prud'homme GJ. Regulation of T-helper-1 versus T-helper-2 activity and enhancement of tumor immunity by combined DNA-based vaccination and nonviral cytokine gene transfer. Gene Ther 2000; 7:481-492.

39. Song K, Chang Y, Prud'homme GJ. IL-12 plasmid-enhanced DNA vaccination against carcinoembryonic antigen (CEA) studied in immune-gene knockout mice. Gene Ther 2000; 7:1527-1535.
40. Estes DM, Brown WC. Type 1 and type 2 responses in regulation of Ig isotype expression in cattle. Vet Immunol Immunopathol 2002; 90:1-10.
41. Davis HL, Brazolot Millan CL, Mancini M et al. DNA-based immunization against hepatitis B surface antigen (HBsAg) in normal and HBsAg-transgenic mice. Vaccine 1997; 15:849-852.
42. Amici A, Smorlesi A, Noce G et al. DNA vaccination with full-length or truncated neu induces protective immunity against the development of spontaneous mammary tumors in HER-2/neu transgenic mice. Gene Ther 2000; 7:703-706.
43. Hawkins WG, Gold JS, Dyall R et al. Immunization with DNA coding for gp100 results in CD4 T-cell independent antitumor immunity. Surgery 2000; 128:273-280.
44. Weber LW, Bowne WB, Wolchok JD et al. Tumor immunity and autoimmunity induced by immunization with homologous DNA. J Clin Invest 1998; 102:1258-64.
45. Djilali-Saiah I, Lapierre P, Vittozi S et al. DNA vaccination breaks tolerance for a neo-self antigen in liver: A transgenic murine model of autoimmune hepatitis. J Immunol 2002; 169:4889-4896.
46. Costagliola S, Many MC, Denef JF et al. Genetic immunization of outbred mice with thyrotropin receptor cDNA provides a model of Graves' disease. J Clin Invest 2000; 105:803-811.
47. Anders HJ, Vielhauer V, Eis V et al. Activation of toll-like receptor-9 induces progression of renal disease in MRL-Fas(lpr) mice. FASEB J 2004; 18:534-536.
48. Gilkeson GS, Ruiz P, Pippen AM et al. Modulation of renal disease in autoimmune NZB/NZW mice by immunization with bacterial DNA. J Exp Med 1996; 183:1389-1397.
49. Waisman A, Ruiz PJ, Hirschberg DL et al. Suppressive vaccination with DNA encoding a variable region gene of the T-cell receptor prevents autoimmune encephalomyelitis and activates Th2 immunity. Nat Med 1996; 2:899-905.
50. Kumar V, Maglione J, Thatte J et al. Induction of a type 1 regulatory CD4 T cell response following V beta 8.2 DNA vaccination results in immune deviation and protection from experimental autoimmune encephalomyelitis. Int Immunol 2001; 13:835-841.
51. Lobell A, Weissert R, Eltayeb S et al. Suppressive DNA vaccination in myelin oligodendrocyte glycoprotein peptide-induced experimental autoimmune encephalomyelitis involves a T1-biased immune response. J Immunol 2003; 170:1806-1813.
52. Prud'homme GJ, Lawson RR, Theofilopoulos AN. Anticytokine gene therapy of autoimmune diseases. Expert Opinion on Biological Therapy 2001; 1:359-373.
53. Tran EH, Prince EN, Owens T. IFN-gamma shapes immune invasion of the central nervous system via regulation of chemokines. J Immunol 2000; 164:2759-2768.
54. Ruiz PJ, Garren H, Ruiz IU et al. Suppressive immunization with DNA encoding a self-peptide prevents autoimmune disease: Modulation of T cell costimulation. J Immunol 1999; 162:3336-3341.
55. Tsunoda I, Kuang LQ, Tolley ND et al. Enhancement of experimental allergic encephalomyelitis (EAE) by DNA immunization with myelin proteolipid protein (PLP) plasmid DNA. J Neuropathol Exp Neurol 1998; 57:758-767.
56. Bourquin C, Iglesias A, Berger T et al. Myelin oligodendrocyte glycoprotein-DNA vaccination induces antibody-mediated autoaggression in experimental autoimmune encephalomyelitis. Eur J Immunol 2000; 30:3663-3671.
57. Selmaj K, Kowal C, Walczak A et al. Naked DNA vaccination differentially modulates autoimmune responses in experimental autoimmune encephalomyelitis. J Neuroimmunol 2000; 111:34-44.
58. Lobell A, Weissert R, Eltayeb S et al. Presence of CpG DNA and the local cytokine milieu determine the efficacy of suppressive DNA vaccination in experimental autoimmune encephalomyelitis. J Immunol 1999; 163:4754-4762.
59. Garren H, Ruiz PJ, Watkins TA et al. Combination of gene delivery and DNA vaccination to protect from and reverse Th1 autoimmune disease via deviation to the Th2 pathway. Immunity 2001; 15:15-22.
60. Genain CP, Abel K, Belmar N et al. Late complications of immune deviation therapy in a nonhuman primate. Science 1996; 274:2054-2057.

61. Weissert R, Lobell A, de Graaf KL et al. Protective DNA vaccination against organ-specific autoimmunity is highly specific and discriminates between single amino acid substitutions in the peptide autoantigen. Proc Natl Acad Sci USA 2000; 97:1689-1694.
62. Lobell A, Weissert R, Storch MK et al. Vaccination with DNA encoding an immunodominant myelin basic protein peptide targeted to Fc of immunoglobulin G suppresses experimental autoimmune encephalomyelitis. J Exp Med 1998; 187:1543-1548.
63. Youssef S, Wildbaum G, Maor G et al. Long-lasting protective immunity to experimental autoimmune encephalomyelitis following vaccination with naked DNA encoding C-C chemokines. J Immunol 1998; 161:3870-3879.
64. Youssef S, Wildbaum G, Karin N. Prevention of experimental autoimmune encephalomyelitis by MIP-1alpha and MCP-1 naked DNA vaccines. J Autoimmun 1999; 13:21-29.
65. Wildbaum G, Westermann J, Maor G et al. A targeted DNA vaccine encoding fas ligand defines its dual role in the regulation of experimental autoimmune encephalomyelitis. J Clin Invest 2000; 106:671-679.
66. Adorini L, Gregori S, Harrison LC. Understanding autoimmune diabetes: Insights from mouse models. Trends Mol Med 2002; 8:31-38.
67. Serreze DV, Leiter EH. Genes and cellular requirements for autoimmune diabetes susceptibility in nonobese diabetic mice. Curr Dir Autoimmun 2001; 4:31-67.
68. Suarez-Pinzon WL, Rabinovitch A. Approaches to type 1 diabetes prevention by intervention in cytokine immunoregulatory circuits. Int J Exp Diabetes Res 2001; 2:3-17.
69. Gottlieb PA, Hayward AR. Cytokine and immunosuppressive therapies of type 1 diabetes mellitus. Endocrinol Metab Clin North Am 2002; 31:477-495.
70. Peakman M, Dayan CM. Antigen-specific immunotherapy for autoimmune disease: Fighting fire with fire? Immunol 2001; 104:361-366.
71. Anderton SM. Peptide-based immunotherapy of autoimmunity: A path of puzzles, paradoxes and possibilities. Immunol 2001; 104:367-376.
72. Simone EA, Wegmann DR, Eisenbarth GS. Immunologic "vaccination" for the prevention of autoimune diabetes (type 1A). Diabetes Care 1999; 22: B7-B15.
73. Bach JF, Chatenoud L. Tolerance to islet autoantigens in type 1 diabetes. Annu Rev Immunol 2001; 19:131-161.
74. Tian J, Olcott A, Hanssen L et al. Antigen-based immunotherapy for autoimmune disease: From animal models to humans? Immunol Today 1999; 20:190-195.
75. Graves PM, Eisenbarth GS. Pathogenesis, prediction and trials for the prevention of insulin-dependent (type 1) diabetes mellitus. Adv Drug Delivery Rev 1999; 35:143-156.
76. Bach JF, Koutouzov S, Van Endert PM. Are there unique autoantigens triggering autoimmune diseases? Immunol Rev 1998; 164:139-155.
77. Bach JF. Immunotherapy to insulin-dependent diabetes mellitus. Curr Opinion Immunol 2001; 13:601-605.
78. Gottlieb PA, Eisenbarth GS. Insulin-specific tolerance in diabetes. Clin Immunol 2002; 102:2-11.
79. Urbanek-Ruiz I, Ruiz PJ, Steinman L et al. Immunomodulatory vaccination in autoimmune disease. Endocrinol Metab Clin North Am 2002; 31:441-456 viii-ix.
80. Sadelain MW, Qin HY, Lauzon J et al. Prevention of type I diabetes in NOD mice by adjuvant immunotherapy. Diabetes 1990; 39:583-589.
81. Shehadeh NN, larosa F, Lafferty KJ. Altered cytokine activity in adjuvant inhibition of autoimmune disease. J Autoimmunity 1993; 6:291-300.
82. Qin HY, Elliott JF, Lakey JRT et al. Endogenous immune response to glutamic acid decarboxylase (GAD67) in NOD mice is modulated by adjuvant immunotherapy. J Autoimmunity 1998; 11:591-601.
83. Elias D, Tikochinski Y, Frankel G et al. Regulation of NOD mouse autoimmune diabetes by T cells that recognize a TCR CDR3 peptide. Int Immunol 1999; 11:957-966.
84. McKeever U, Khandekar S, Newcomb J et al. Immunization with soluble BDC 2.5 T cell receptor-immunoglobulin chimeric protein: Antibody specificity and protection of nonobese diabetic mice against adoptive transfer of diabetes by maternal immunization. J Exp Med 1996; 184:1755-1768.

85. Allen HF, Klingensmith GJ, Jensen P et al. Effect of Bacillus Calmette-Guerin vaccination on new-onset type 1 diabetes. A randomized clinical study. Diabetes Care 1999; 22:1703-7.
86. Tian J, Olcott AP, Hanssen LR et al. Infectious Th1 and Th2 autoimmunity in diabetes-prone mice. Immunol Rev 1998; 164:119-127.
87. Yoon JW, Yoon CS, Lim HW et al. Control of autoimmune diabetes in NOD mice by GAD expression or suppression in beta cells. Science 1999; 284:1183-1187.
88. Geng L, Solimena M, Flavell RA et al. Widespread expression of an autoantigen-GAD65 transgene does not tolerize nonobese diabetic mice and can exacerbate disease. Proc Natl Acad Sci USA 1998; 95:10055-10060.
89. Bridgett M, Cetkovic-Cvrlje M, O'Rourke R et al. Differential protection in two transgenic lines of NOD/Lt mice hyperexpressing the autoantigen GAD65 in pancreatic beta-cells. Diabetes 1998; 47:1848-1856.
90. Kash SF, Condie BG, Baekkeskov S. Glutamate decarboxylase and GABA in pancreatic islets: Lessons from knockout mice. Hormone Metab Res 1999; 31:340-344.
91. Tisch R, Wang B, Serreze DV. Induction of glutamic acid decarboxylase 65-specific Th2 cells and suppression of autoimmune diabetes at late stages of disease is epitope dependent. J Immunol 1999; 163:1178-1187.
92. Wang B, Gonzalez A, Hoglund P et al. Interleukin-4 deficiency does not exacerbate disease in NOD mice. Diabetes 1998; 47:1207-1211.
93. Katz JD, Benoist C, Mathis D. T helper cell subsets in insulin-dependent diabetes. Science 1995; 268:1185-1188.
94. Suri A, Katz JD. Dissecting the role of CD4+ T cells in autoimmune diabetes through the use of TCR transgenic mice. Immunol Rev 1999; 169:55-65.
95. Tarbell KV, Lee M, Ranheim E et al. CD4+ T cells from glutamic acid decarboxylase (GAD)65-specific T cell receptor transgenic mice are not diabetogenic and can delay diabetes transfer. J Exp Med 2002; 196:481-492.
96. Polanski M, Melican NS, Zhang J et al. Oral administration of the immunodominant B-chain of insulin reduces diabetes in a cotransfer modes of diabetes in the NOD mouse and is associated with a switch from Th1 to Th2 cytokines. J Autoimmunity 1997; 10:339-346.
97 Harrison LC, Dempsey-Collier M, Kramer DR et al. Aerosol insulin induces regulatory CD8 gamma/delta T cells that prevent murine insulin-dependent diabetes. J Exp Med 1996; 184:2167-2174.
98 Ramiya VK, Shang XZ, Wasserfall CH et al. Effect of oral and intravenous insulin and glutamic acid decarboxylase in NOD mice. Autoimmunity 1997; 26:139-151.
99. Hutchings P, Cooke A. Comparative study of the protective effect afforded by intravenous administration of bovine or ovine insulin to young NOD mice. Diabetes 1995; 44:906-910.
100. Daniel D, Wegmann DR. Protection of nonobese diabetic mice from diabetes by intranasal or subcutaneous administration of insulin B-(9-23). Proc Natl Acad Sci USA 1996; 93:956-960.
101. Chen W, Bergerot I, Elliott JF et al. Evidence that a peptide spanning the B-C junction of proinsulin I is an early autoantigen epitope in the pathogenesis of type 1 diabetes. J Immunol 2001; 167: 4926-4935.
102. Wegmann DR, Norbury-Glaser M, Daniel D. Insulin-specific T-cells are a predominant component of islet infiltrates in prediabetic NOD mice. Eur J Immunol 1994; 24:1853-1857.
103. Wong FS, Karttunen J, Dumont C et al. Identification of an MHC class I-restricted autoantigen in type 1 diabetes by screening an organ-specific cDNA library. Nature Med 1999; 5:1026-1031.
104. Daniel D, Gill RG, Schloot N et al. Epitope specificity, cytokine production profile and diabetogenic activity of insulin-specific T cell clones isolated from NOD mice. Eur J Immunol 1995; 25:056-1062.
105. Simone EA, Yu L, Wegmann DR et al. T cell receptor gene polymorphysisms associated with anti-insulin, autoimmune T cells in diabetes-prone NOD mice. J Autoimmunity 1997; 10:317-321.
106. Trentham DE. Oral tolerization as a treatment of rheumatoid arthritis. Rheumatic Diseases Clinics of North America 1998; 24:525-536.
107. Quintana FJ, Rotem A, Carmi P et al. Vaccination with empty plasmid DNA or CpG oligonucleotide inhibits diabetes in nonobese diabetic mice: Modulation of spontaneous 60-kDa heat shock protein autoimmunity. J Immunol 2000; 165:6148-6155.

108. Quintana FJ, Carmi P, Cohen IR. DNA vaccination with heat shock protein 60 inhibits cyclophosphamide-accelerated diabetes. J Immunol 2002; 169:6030-6035.
109. Coon B, An LL, Whitton Jl et al. DNA immunization to prevent autoimmune diabetes. J Clin Invest 1999; 104:189-194.
110. Karges W, Pechhold K, Al Dahouk S et al. Induction of autoimmune diabetes through insulin (but not GAD65) DNA vaccination in nonobese diabetic and in RIP-B7.1 mice. Diabetes 2002; 51:3237-3244.
111. Urbanek-Ruiz I, Ruiz PJ, Paragas V et al. Immunization with DNA encoding an immunodominant peptide of insulin prevents diabetes in NOD mice. Clin Immunol 2001; 100:164-171.
112. Bot A, Smith D, Bot S et al. Plasmid vaccination with insulin B chain prevents autoimmune diabetes in nonobese diabetic mice. J Immunol 2001; 167:2950-2955.
113. Weaver Jr DJ, Liu B, Tisch R. Plasmid DNAs encoding insulin and glutamic acid decarboxylase 65 have distinct effects on the progression of autoimmune diabetes in nonobese diabetic mice. J Immunol 2001; 167:586-592.
114. Wiest-Ladenburger U, Fortnagel A, Richter W et al. DNA vaccination with glutamic acid decarboxylase (GAD) generates a strong humoral immune response in BALB/c, C57BL/6, and in diabetes-prone NOD mice. Horm Metab Res 1998; 30:605-609.
115. Balasa B, Boehm BO, Fortnagel A et al. Vaccination with glutamic acid decarboxylase plasmid DNA protects mice from spontaneous autoimmune diabetes and B7/CD28 costimulation circumvents that protection. Clin Immunol 2001; 99:241-252.
116. Jun HS, Chung YH, Han J et al. Prevention of autoimmune diabetes by immunogene therapy using recombinant vaccinia virus expressing glutamic acid decarboxylase. Diabetologia 2002; 45:668-676.
117. Glinka Y, de Pooter R, Croze F et al. Regulatory cytokine production stimulated by DNA vaccination against an altered form of glutamic acid decarboxylase 65 (GAD65) in nonobese diabetic (NOD) mice. J Mol Med 2003 In press.
118. Groux H, O'Garra A, Bigler M et al. A CD4+ T-cell subset inhibits antigen-specific T-cell responses and prevents colitis. Nature 1997; 389:737-742.
119. Shevach E. Regulatory T cells in autoimmmunity. Annu Rev Immunol 2000; 18:423-449.
120. Shevach E, McHugh R, Piccirillo C et al. Control of T-cell activation by CD4+ CD25+ suppressor T cells. Immunol Rev 2001; 182:58-67.
121. Filippova M, Liu J, Escher A. Effects of plasmid DNA injection on cyclophosphamide-accelerated diabetes in NOD mice. DNA Cell Biol 2001; 20:175-181.
122. Tarbell KV, Lee M, Ranheim E et al. CD4(+) T cells from glutamic acid decarboxylase (GAD)65-specific T cell receptor transgenic mice are not diabetogenic and can delay diabetes transfer. J Exp Med 2002; 196:481-492.
123. Dieckmann D, Bruett C, Ploettner H et al. Human CD4(+)CD25(+) regulatory, contact-dependent T cells induce interleukin 10-producing, contact-independent type 1-like regulatory T cells. J Exp Med 2002; 196:247-253.
124. Moore K, de Waal M, Coffman R et al. Interleukin-10 and the interleukin-10 receptor. Annu Rev Immunol 2001; 19:683-765.
125. Prud'homme GJ, Chang Y. Prevention of autoimmune diabetes by intramuscular gene therapy with a nonviral vector encoding an interferon-gamma receptor/IgG1 fusion protein. Gene Ther 1999; 6:771-777.
126. Chang Y, Prud'homme GJ. Intramuscular administration of expression plasmids encoding interferon-gamma-receptor/IgG1 or IL-4/IgG1 chimeric proteins protects from autoimmunity. J Gene Med 1999; 1:415-423.
127. Schloot N, Hanifi-Moghaddam P, Goebel C et al. Serum IFN-gamma and IL-10 levels are associated with disease progression in nonobese diabetic mice. Diabetes Metab Res Rev 2002; 18:64-70.
128. Freeman G, Sharpe A, Kuchroo V. Protect the killer: CTLs need defenses against the tumor. Nat Med 2002; 8:787-789.
129. Pennline K, Roque-Gaffney E, Monahan M. Recombinant human IL-10 prevents the onset of diabetes in the nonobese diabetic mouse. Clin Immunol Immunopathol 1994; 71:169-175.

130. Zheng X, Steele A, Hancock W et al. A noncytolytic IL-10/Fc fusion protein prevents diabetes, blocks autoimmunity, and promotes suppressor phenomena in NOD mice. J Immunol 1997; 158:4507-4513.
131. Moritani M, Yoshimoto K, Ii S et al. Prevention of adoptively transferred diabetes in nonobese diabetic mice with IL-10-transduced islet-specific Th1 lymphocytes. A gene therapy model for autoimmune diabetes. J Clin Invest 1996; 98:1851-1859.
132. Piccirillo C, Chang Y, Prud'homme GJ. TGF-beta1 somatic gene therapy prevents autoimmune disease in nonobese diabetic mice. J Immunol 1998; 161:3950-3956.
133. Wolfe T, Bot A, Hughes A et al. Endogenous expression levels of autoantigens influence success or failure of DNA immunizations to prevent type 1 diabetes: Addition of IL-4 increases safety. Eur J Immunol 2002; 32:113-121.
134. Hartikka J, Sawdey M, Cornefert-Jensen F et al. An improved plasmid DNA expression vector for direct injection into skeletal muscle. Hum Gene Ther 1996; 7:1205-1217.
135. Tisch R, Wang B, Weaver DJ et al. Antigen-specific mediated suppression of beta cell autoimmunity by plasmid DNA vaccination. J Immunol 2001; 166:2122-2132.
136. Chambers CA, Kuhns MS, Egen JG et al. CTLA-4-mediated inhibition in regulation of immune responses: Mechanisms and manipulation in tumor immunotherapy. Ann Rev Immunol 2001; 19:565-594.
137. Salomon B, Bluestone JA. Complexities of CD28/B7: CTLA-4 costimulatory pathways in autoimmunity and transplantation. Ann Rev Immunol 2001; 19:225-252.
138. Dahlen E, Hedlund G, Dawe K. Low CD86 expression in the nonobese diabetic mouse results in impairment of both T cell activation and CTLA-4 up-regulation. J Immunol 2000; 164:2444-2456.
139. Awata T, Kurihara S, Iitaka M et al. Association of CTLA-4 A-G polymorphism (IDDM12 locus) with acute onset and insulin-depleted IDDM as well as autoimmune thyroiditis (Graves' disease and Hashimoto thyroiditis) in the Japanese population. Diabetes 1998; 47:128-129.
140. Kouki T, Sawai Y, Gardine CA et al. CTLA-4 gene polymorphism at position 49 in exon 1 reduces the inhibitory function of CTLA-4 and contributes to the pathogenesis of Graves' disease. J Immunol 2000; 165:6606-6611.
141. Luhder F, Chambers C, Allison JP et al. Pinpointing when T cell costimulatory receptor CTLA-4 must be engaged to dampen diabetogenic T cell. Proc Natl Acad Sci USA 2000; 97:12204-12209.
142. Piganelli JD, Poulin M, Martin T et al. Cytotoxic T lymphocyte antigen 4 (CD152) regulates self-reactive T cells in BALB/c but not in autoimmune NOD mouse. J Autoimmun 2000; 14:123-131.
143. Takahashi T, Tagami T, Yamazaki S et al. Immunologic tolerance maintained by CD25+CD4+ regulatory T cells constitutively expressing cytotoxic T lymphoycte-associated antigen 4. J Exp Med 2000; 192:303-310.
144. Salomon B, Lenschow DJ, Rhee L et al. B7/CD28 costimulation is essential for the homeostasis of the CD4+CD25+ immunoregulatory T cells that control autoimmune diabetes. Immunity 2000; 12:431-440.
145. Read S, Malmstrom V, Powrie F. Cytotoxic T lymphocyte-associated antigen 4 plays an essential role in the function of CD25+ CD4+ regulatory cells that control intestinal inflammation. J Exp Med 2000; 192:295-302.
146. Chen W, Jin W, Wahl SM. Engagement of cytotoxic T lymphocyte antigen 4 (CTLA-4) induces transforming growth factor beta (TGF-beta) production by murine CD4+ T cells. J Exp Med 1998; 188:1849-1857.
147. Saverino D, Merlo A, Bruno S et al. Dual effect of CD85/leukocyte Ig-like receptor-1/Ig-like transcript 2 and CD152 (CTLA-4) on cytokine production by antigen-stimulated human T cells. J Immunol 2002; 168:207-215.
148. Gomes NA, Gattass CR, Barreto-De-Souza V et al. TGF-beta mediates CTLA-4 suppression of cellular immunity in murine kalaazar. J Immunol 2000; 164:2001-2008.
149. Guo Y, Wu Y, Kong X et al. Identification of conserved amino acids in murine B7-1IgV domain critical for CTLA4/CD28:B7 interaction by site-directed mutagenesis: A novel structural model of the binding site. Mol Immunol 1998; 35:215-225.
150. Guo Y, Wu Y, Zhao M et al. Mutational analysis of an alternatively spliced product of B7 defines its CD28/CTLA4-binding site on immunoglobulin C domain. J Exp Med 1995; 181:1345-1355.

151. Prud'homme GJ, Chang Y, Li X. Immunoinhibitory DNA vaccine protects against autoimmune diabetes through cDNA encoding a selective CTLA-4 (CD152) ligand. Hum Gene Ther 2002; 13:395-406.
152. Argeas CA, Truneh A, Reddy M et al. Identification of residues in the V domain of CD80 (B7-1) implicated in functional interactions with CD28 and CTLA-4. J Exp Med 1995; 182:667-675.
153. Ragno S, Colston MJ, Lowrie DB et al. Protection of rats from adjuvant arthritis by immunization with naked DNA encoding for mycobacterial heat shock protein 65. Arthritis Rheum 1997; 40:277-283.
154. Youssef S, Maor G, Wildbaum G et al. C-C chemokine–encoding DNA vaccines enhance breakdown of tolerance to their gene products and treat ongoing adjuvant arthritis. J Clin Invest 2000; 106:361-371.
155. Wildbaum G, Youssef S, Karin N. A targeted DNA vaccine augments the natural immune response to self TNF-alpha and suppresses ongoing adjuvant arthritis. J Immunol 2000; 165:5860-5866.
156. Matsumoto Y, Jee Y, Sugisaki M. Successful TCR-based immunotherapy for autoimmune myocarditis with DNA vaccines after rapid identification of pathogenic TCR. J Immunol 2000; 164:2248-2254.
157. Fan GC, Singh RR. Vaccination with minigenes encoding V(H)-derived major histocompatibility complex class I-binding epitopes activates cytotoxic T cells that ablate autoantibody-producing B cells and inhibit lupus. J Exp Med 2002; 196:731-741.
158. Kitagaki K, Jain VV, Businga TR et al. Immunomodulatory effects of CpG oligodeoxynucleotides on established Th2 responses. Clin Diagn Lab Immunol 2002; 9:1260-1269.
159. Yi AK, Yoon JG, Yeo SJ et al. Role of mitogen-activated protein kinases in CpG DNA-mediated IL-10 and IL-12 production: Central role of extracellular signal-regulated kinase in the negative feedback loop of the CpG DNA-mediated Th1 response. J Immunol 2002; 168:4711-4720.
160. Pasare C, Medzhitov R. Toll pathway-dependent blockade of CD4+CD25+ T cell-mediated suppression by dendritic cells. Science 2003; 299:1033-1036.

Index

L

M

N

O

P

R

S

T

V

MIX
Papier aus verantwortungsvollen Quellen
Paper from responsible sources
FSC® C105338

If you have any concerns about our products,
you can contact us on
ProductSafety@springernature.com

In case Publisher is established outside the EU,
the EU authorized representative is:
Springer Nature Customer Service Center GmbH
Europaplatz 3, 69115 Heidelberg, Germany

Printed by Libri Plureos GmbH
in Hamburg, Germany